Official
Guide to
OET®

Special thanks to the team who made this book possible:

Cat Ahlberg, Edward Antram, Kim Bowers, Louise Cook, Lindsey Dew, Scarlet Edmonds, Joanna Graham, Brad Hissey, Brian Holmes, Sirkka Howes, Amna Hussein, Eleanor Lindberg, Nimesh Shah, David Wiltshire, Kevin Yang, Amy Zarkos

Published by Kaplan Publishing, a division of Kaplan, Inc.
750 Third Avenue
New York, NY 10017

ISBN: 978-1-5062-4724-3

10 9 8 7 6 5 4 3 2 1

Kaplan Publishing books are available at special quantity discounts to use for sales promotions, employee premiums, or educational purposes. For more information or to purchase books, please call the Simon & Schuster special sales department at 1-866-506-1949.

TABLE OF
CONTENTS

How to Use This Book vii

GO ONLINE

*www.kaptest.com/
booksonline*

PART ONE: **The Basics**. 1

Chapter 1: **Taking OET** 3

  Understanding OET 3

  An Overview of OET 4

Chapter 2: **Preparing for Test Day**. 7

  Study Planner. 7

  OET Study Planner. 8

  OET Study Planner 9

  General Strategies for OET 10

  Tips for the Final Week. 10

PART TWO: **The Listening Section** 13

Listening Introduction 15

  Section Overview. 15

Chapter 3: **Listening Part A** 17

  Strategies 17

  Part A Practice Set 23

  Answers 25

  Listening Transcripts. 27

Chapter 4: **Listening Part B** 31

  Strategies 32

  Part B Practice Set 37

  Answers 38

  Listening Transcripts. 39

Table of Contents

Chapter 5: **Listening Part C** 45

Strategies 45

Part C Practice Set 50

Answers 53

Listening Transcripts 54

PART THREE: **The Reading Section** 59

Reading Introduction 61

Section Overview 61

Chapter 6: **Reading Part A** 63

Strategies 63

Part A Practice Set 75

Answers 82

Chapter 7: **Reading Part B** 85

Strategies 85

Part B Practice Set 96

Answers 102

Chapter 8: **Reading Part C** 103

Strategies 103

Part C Practice Set 111

Answers 118

PART FOUR: **The Writing Section** 119

Writing Introduction 121

Section Overview 121

Chapter 9: **The Writing Task** 123

Strategies 124

Writing Practice Set 137

Answers 145

PART FIVE: **The Speaking Section** 153

Speaking Introduction 155

Section Overview 155

Chapter 10: **The Speaking Task** 157

   Strategies 157

   Speaking Practice Set 171

   Answers 179

PART SIX: **The Practice Test** 181

   OET: **Listening Section** 183

      Part A 183

      Part B 185

      Part C 187

   OET: **Reading Section** 189

      Part A 189

      Part B 194

      Part C 200

   OET: **Writing Section** 209

   OET: **Speaking Section** 215

      Answers 223

      Listening Scripts 229

How to Use This Book

This book has been created to help you achieve the highest possible score in OET. Each part includes easy-to-learn strategies and relevant test-taking tips. There's also a weekly study planner, access to listening tracks, sample writing answers, and a full length Practice Test with Writing and Speaking specific to the Nursing and Medicine healthcare professions. Follow the steps below to get the best use from this book.

Step One: Read Part One

In the first part of this book, you will be given an overview of OET, learn what to expect on Test Day, and learn about the key strategies to help you achieve a high OET score.

Step Two: Fill Out Your Study Planner

OET is a high stakes test. If you want to score well, you cannot squeeze all of your study time into one week. Before getting started with the exercises in this book, you should turn to Part 2 and fill out your study planner with realistic study goals. You should consider how many days you have until you take OET, and how much time you will realistically be able to dedicate to revising every day. Remember that if you have worked all day, you may not have the energy to learn new strategies. Instead, use the time to revise the parts of the test you have already mastered, and save the more challenging parts for when you are fresh and rested.

Step Three: Sharpen Your Skills

This book contains exercises and strategies for correctly answering each section of OET. The most important strategies for your success are highlighted, so you can easily refer to them. At the end of each section, you will find practice questions.

Once you have completed the questions, turn to the answers and mark your work. Check through any incorrect answers, using the listening scripts at the back of the chapter if needed.

Step Four: Use the Online Audio

Part Two and the full length Practice Test at the end of this book include audio. Register online at **kaptest.com/booksonline** to access your audio and online resources. Once you've registered, access your audio and resources at kaptest.com/login or download the Kaplan Mobile Prep app on Google Play or the App Store for your Android or iOS device.

Step Five: Take Kaplan's OET Practice Test

After practising the strategies for OET, you should use the Practice Test as a test run for the real thing. After taking the test, use the answer key to score the Listening and Reading sections of your Practice Test, and use the marking criteria for the Speaking and Writing sections to grade your work.

Step Six: Review

Return to Parts Two, Three, Four and Five of this book, and review those sections of the test where your performance was weak. Read the Tips for the Final Week to make sure you are fully prepared on Test Day.

Follow these six steps, and you can be confident that you are truly ready for OET.

PART ONE

The Basics

CHAPTER 1

Taking OET

IN THIS CHAPTER

- Understanding OET
- How and Where OET is administered
- An Overview of OET
- Filling Out the Answer Sheet

Understanding OET

Before getting started with the content of OET, let's look at some background information about the test.

What is OET?

The Occupational English Test (OET) was developed to test healthcare professionals' English communication abilities. OET tests English language ability in four areas: Listening, Reading, Writing and Speaking. Test-takers will need to demonstrate their ability to understand and answer questions about general healthcare consultations and presentations, in addition to texts in a general healthcare setting. Test-takers are required to write accurate, professional letters with the aid of prompts and use speaking prompts to carry out appropriate and effective conversations with patients, relating to specific healthcare professions.

Who Produces OET?

OET was developed by Professor Tim McNamara at the University of Melbourne. It has been owned and produced by Cambridge Box Hill Language Assessment Trust – a venture between Cambridge English and Box Hill Institute – since 2013.

Which Version of OET?

OET can be taken by healthcare professions in any of the following 12 professions: Dentistry, Dietetics, Medicine, Nursing, Occupational Therapy, Optometry, Pharmacy, Physiotherapy, Podiatry, Radiography, Speech Pathology, and Veterinary Science.

The Reading and Listening parts of this book are relevant to all 12 healthcare professions. The Speaking and Writing parts of this book cover Nursing and Medicine specific test content. Please note that if you are a healthcare professional from a different profession, the Speaking and Writing sections of your test will vary from the content provided in this book.

When was OET Updated

In September 2018, Cambridge Boxhill Language Assessment launched an updated format of OET in the Reading and Listening sections of the text, to more accurately assess the English language abilities of test-takers in a healthcare setting, and create additional assessment criteria for the Speaking Test. This book discusses the 2018 OET test format.

How to apply for OET?

You can apply to take OET by visiting www.occupationalenglishtest.org/apply-oet/. When you register to take OET, you might only be able to select from the next two available test dates, so you should aim to begin revising for the test before applying. To apply online, you will need to refer to an identification document and upload a colour passport photograph of yourself.

An Overview of OET

Format and Content

OET is approximately 2 hours and 45 minutes long and consists of 42 Listening questions, 42 Reading questions, 2 Speaking role-plays and 1 Writing task. The following chart gives a breakdown of the times for each part of OET

Test Section	Time	Tests candidate's ability to
Listening	40 minutes	listen and understand a range of recordings on healthcare topics from different healthcare settings.
Reading	60 minutes	read and understand various texts on healthcare topics from different healthcare settings.
Writing	45 minutes	write a letter, usually a referral letter using information provided in patient case notes.
Speaking	20 minutes	communicate with a patient in a real-life context through the use of role-plays.

Scoring

In OET, candidates receive a numerical score ranging from 0 to 500 in ten-point increments (e.g. 350, 360, 370…). The numerical scores will be mapped to a separate letter grade for each section of the test, ranging from A (highest) to E (lowest). There is no overall grade.

OET results to August 2018	OET scores from September 2018	OET band descriptors	IELTS equivalent band score
A	500 490 480 470 460 450	Can communicate very fluently and effectively with patients and health professionals using appropriate register, tone and lexis. Shows complete understanding of any kind of written or spoken language	8.0 – 9.0
B	440 430 420 410 400 390 380 370 360 350	Can communicate effectively with patients and health professionals using appropriate register, tone and lexis, with only occasional inaccuracies and hesitations. Shows good understanding in a range of clinical contexts.	7.5 – 7.0
C+	340 330 320 310 300	Can maintain the interaction in a relevant healthcare environment despite occasional errors and lapses, and follow standard spoken language normally encountered in his/her field of specialisation.	6.5
C	290 280 270 260 250 240 230 220 210 200		6.0 – 5.5

(Continued)

OET results to August 2018	OET scores from September 2018	OET band descriptors	IELTS equivalent band score
D	190 180 170 160 150 140 130 120 110 100	Can maintain some interaction and understand straightforward factual information in his/her filed of speciali-sation, but may ask for clarification. Frequent errors, inaccuracies and mis- or overuse of technical language can cause strain in communication.	Less than 5.5
E	90 80 70 60 50 40 30 20 10 0	Can manage simple interaction on familiar topics and understand the main point in short, simple messages, provided he/she can ask for clarifica-tion. High density of error and mis- or overuse of technical language cause significant strain and breakdowns in communication.	

Timing

OET is a timed test. This means that your score greatly depends on being able to complete the questions within the time allowed.

We will indicate the amount of time you will be given to complete each part of the test at the beginning of each chapter. In the Listening Test, you will not need to time yourself, as you will be advised when to answer questions while you listen to the recording, but you will still need to keep up with the pace of the recording. At first, you may not feel you have enough time to answer the questions and complete the tasks effectively. However, by practising the strategies in this book, you should be able to get through all of the test questions in the time provided. Remember that even if you are not able to complete a whole section within the time limit, you should still include an answer – even if it is a guess – on your answer sheet. You may choose the correct answer by chance, and gain an additional point; if you leave those questions unanswered, you will receive no points.

As you go through the book, pay attention to the amount of time you spend answering questions and completing tasks; note when you are moving too slowly, and practise speaking, writing and answering questions more quickly. When you are ready to take the Practice Test, be sure to time yourself very carefully, to give yourself the most realistic test experience possible, and to show you exactly where you need improvement.

CHAPTER 2

Preparing for Test Day

IN THIS CHAPTER

- Study Planner
- General strategies for OET
- Tips for the final week
- Stress busters

Study Planner

On the next two pages, you will find a couple of five-week calendars. Use these calendars to fill in a specific study schedule. Be realistic about the amount of time you have to study and practise your English language skills. Update your schedule as necessary.

Do not forget to schedule time to take the Practice Test, mark your Practice Test, and review any part of the test where you struggled along with your schedule for looking through the rest of the book. Take the Practice Test after you have looked at all of the other chapters of the book and completed all of the exercises. Take the Practice Test as if it were the real thing: find a quiet place where you will not be interrupted, and take it in one session. Time yourself accurately. This will help to prepare you for the actual test.

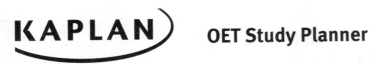

OET Study Planner

Month:_____

Monday	Tuesday	Wednesday	Thursday	Friday	Saturday	Sunday

To do this month:

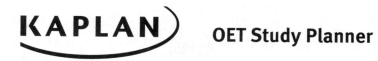 **OET Study Planner**

Month:_____

Monday	Tuesday	Wednesday	Thursday	Friday	Saturday	Sunday

To do this month:

General Strategies for OET

Look through the tips in this section to make sure you are aware of the practical steps you should take before Test Day. This section also contains tips on how and how often to revise. All OET test takers are already familiar with high pressure test situations, but each test is different, and requires different preparation and materials, so make sure you're aware of what you need to do before you take the test.

Tips for the Final Week

In the week before your test, you should do the following:

- Recheck your registration for accuracy; contact the OET helpdesk if there are any problems.
- Visit the test venue if possible. It can be helpful to know how long it takes you to get there, and to see the test venue where you will actually take your test.
- Practise working on test material as if it were Test Day.
- Look at your results from the Practice Test and content in this book, and identify your strengths and weaknesses. Use the last week before Test Day to focus on your weaker areas, and reread those chapters of this book.

The Day Before Test Day

Try to avoid doing intensive studying the day before the test. As healthcare professionals, you are likely revising for the test alongside a busy work schedule. On the day before the test, you are likely to already know all you need to about taking OET. Instead of trying to learn new information, you might find it helpful to review key strategies, prepare everything you will need for Test Day, and try to find some free time to relax.

Test Day

Plan to arrive early at your test venue; the administrators will not admit latecomers. Make sure you have your test kit with you, especially your ID.

During the test, try not to think about how you are performing. Instead, focus on the task of providing the correct answer, reading and listening actively, and speaking and writing clearly. Think about how well you have prepared, and be confident and positive about your abilities.

After OET

After all your hard work in preparing for OET, be sure to celebrate once it is over. Get together with your family and friends, relax, and have fun. You have a lot to celebrate: You prepared for the test ahead of time. You did your best. You've done all you can to get a good score.

Before the Test

As a qualified health professional, you are already used to revising for and passing difficult tests, and dealing with stress. However, OET is an English language test, and will require you to prepare in a slightly different way than the previous tests you have encountered. Here are some tips for preparing yourself ahead of your test, so you can perform well on Test Day.

Make English a Part of Every Day

Surround yourself with the English language in the weeks and months leading up to your test. Get in the habit of reading or listening to something in English every day, and writing and speaking in English about what you have learned. These activities should be completed separately from your study time. Even just half an hour of practising each day will help you to improve you general English skills. Even more importantly, you will become more and more familiar, and therefore more comfortable, with English. The level of comfort you have with English, whether you are listening, reading, writing or speaking, will help reduce stress and nervousness when you take OET.

Talk

Talk to friends or colleagues who are taking OET, or have already taken it. Sharing your strategies, and hearing their experiences with revising for and taking the test will help you to get ready for Test Day. Remember there isn't one strategy that will work for everyone. Try the strategies suggested by your friends and colleagues but also feel confident to develop your own or to use the ones suggested in this book. If you do discuss OET with colleagues who have already taken OET, remember that the format of the test has changed over the years, so make sure to check www.occupationalenglishtest.org to confirm that you know what to expect for your test.

Take a Break

Remember that in order to learn something, it is necessary to give yourself a break every so often, to allow your mind to process new information. Healthcare professionals are used to working long shifts, and absorbing large amounts of factual information, but improving language requires a different approach. Make sure you give yourself time to have a break, from both OET revision and work. The easiest way to do this is to start revising at the earliest opportunity, so that you have enough time to read through all of the information in this book, and still give yourself time to relax.

During the Test

OET requires a high level of concentration and quick responses. Your state of mind as you take the test will affect your score. Here are some tips for performing your best as you take OET.

Keep Moving

When you find yourself stuck during OET, whether you're struggling to understand what a speaker is saying in the Listening Test, trying to find meaning in a difficult paragraph in the Reading Test, or trying to remember the correct word or phrase to use in the Speaking and Writing Tests, remind yourself that it is okay to make some mistakes on OET. You do not have to get everything right to achieve a good score, so do not spend an excessive amount of time on a question that is too difficult for you, or trying to remember a phrase to use. Make an educated guess, or explain what you mean as best you can, and then move on!

Concentrate

Other test takers may seem to be working more busily than you are, but do not pay attention to them! Other people's activity levels are not necessarily signs of progress or higher scores. Continue to work carefully and thoroughly, and aim to answer the questions within the time limit.

Think Positively!

While taking OET, remind yourself:

- You do not have to get every single question right to achieve a high score.
- By having studied the strategies in this book, you are better prepared than the majority of other test takers.
- You are probably doing better than you realise.

PART TWO

The Listening Section

Listening Introduction

Section Overview

The OET Listening Test consists of three separate parts with a total of 42 questions, and lasts around 40 minutes. You only hear each recording once, so you should familiarise yourself with the format of each of the three separate parts in this section before Test Day. All of the listening content is appropriate for healthcare professionals in any of the 12 different professions, and does not require specialist knowledge in a particular healthcare field, though the listening content tests your level of English in a healthcare-specific environment.

The three different parts of the Listening Test are described below.

In Part A you hear two different consultations in each of which a healthcare professional is talking to a patient. There is one note-completion task with 12 gaps to fill for each consultation. Part A lasts around 10 minutes and tests your ability to understand and record specific information about patients.

In Part B you hear six different extracts from the workplace. In each extract, you hear healthcare professionals either talking to each other, or to a patient. There is one multiple-choice question to answer about each extract. This Part lasts around ten minutes and tests your ability to understand everyday workplace interaction.

In Part C you hear two longer recordings. Each recording is either an interview or a workplace presentation on a topic related to healthcare. There are six multiple-choice questions to answer about each recording. This part lasts around 15 minutes and tests your ability to understand the speaker's ideas and experiences related to the topic.

Before each recording, you hear information about the context and instructions about what you have to do. This information will also be printed on your test paper. Before each recording, you have time to read through the questions and think about what you're going to hear before you answer the questions.

Listening Strategies

- The OET Listening Test is a fixed format test with standardised instructions. The instructions you see in this book are the instructions you will receive on Test Day. You should make sure you are familiar with these instructions, so you know what to expect ahead of your test.

- The topics in the Listening Test are of generic healthcare interest, accessible to candidates across all professions.

- Use the time you are given before each task in the Listening Test to look at the questions and think about what you're going to hear. You can use this information in Part A and C to help you understand the structure of the recording you will hear, and in Part B, you should read through the questions so that you know what information and ideas you're listening for when you hear the recording.

- You may find it helpful to underline important words in the question for Multiple-Choice questions, and underline important words that appear before and after the gaps in Note Completion questions.

- You only hear the recording for the tasks in the Listening Test once, so you will need to record your answers as you listen.

- Make sure you fill in all of the gaps in Part A, and select an answer choice for all of the questions in Parts B and C. You will not lose marks for incorrect answers.

- Don't worry if you miss an answer as you work through the task – continue to move forward with the recording, otherwise you will miss the next question, too. Once you've finished the task, you can look back at the question you missed, select the answer that seems most likely, and move on.

- Listen to English every day. You can improve your listening abilities by listening to a range of listening materials from a variety of sources, such as podcasts and videos, rather than focusing on test-related contexts.

- Write clearly and legibly – if the assessor can't read what you have written, your answer won't be marked as correct.

Listening Part A

Introduction

In Part A of the Listening Test of OET, you listen to 2 separate consultations and complete notes that follow the details of the consultation, by filling in the gaps. There are 12 gaps for each consultation.

Each consultation in Part A lasts for 4 to 5 minutes. You have 30 seconds to look through the notes before the recording begins, and you must answer the questions as you listen to the consultation.

Strategies

Know the Instructions

You should make sure you are familiar with what you have to do before you take the test. The instructions look like this:

Listening Test

The Listening test has three parts. In each part you'll hear a number of different extracts.

You'll hear each extract **ONCE ONLY**.

Part A

In this part of the test, you'll hear two different extracts. In each extract, a health professional is talking to a patient.

For questions 1 to 24, complete the notes with information you hear in the recording.

Extract 1: Questions 1 to 12

You hear a neurosurgeon talking to a referred patient called Haley Waterman. For **questions 1 to 12**, complete the notes with a word or short phrase.

Know the Format

The consultations you hear in Part A are between a healthcare professional and a patient. Occasionally, the healthcare professional talks with a relative of the patient, instead of the patient themselves. The patient speaks more than the healthcare professional and most of the information in the notes comes from what the patient says.

The consultation between the two speakers covers a number of aspects of the patient's condition and treatment. You should use the 30 seconds of silence before the Part A conversation begins to read the notes and think about the information that you're listening for.

Read the Notes Before the Recording Begins

On Test Day, you have 30 seconds to read through the notes for each Part A consultation before the recording begins. Use this time wisely, to make sure that when the recording begins, you are anticipating the type of information you need to listen for to fill the gaps, such as a symptom, a form of medication or a type of treatment.

As you look through the notes, make sure to consider the following points:

1. What is the structure of the consultation?

Look at the headings and sub-headings in the notes to understand the order of the information you are going to hear. This will help you to follow the recording as you listen, and keep your place in the task.

2. What type of information is needed in the gap?

Look at the notes and think about the type of information that is missing. For example, if the notes before the gap say that symptoms are 'described as' something, this tells you that you're listening for the patient's actual words so that's what you should listen for.

Identifying important information in the notes

Some of the information in the notes will assist your understanding of what type of information you need to complete the blanks. For example, if the notes say 'patient diagnosed with (1)_____ after reporting extreme back pain', the important words are 'diagnosed with', which suggests that you need to listen out for a particular condition, and 'extreme back pain and numbness', which are the symptoms you need to listen out for in the patient's speech. From the information in the notes, we can predict that the patient could say something like:

> *I went to the doctor's because I was having this <u>really terrible pain in my back</u>, and also this <u>numbness</u> in my legs. After doing some tests, <u>they said I had</u> **sciatica.**

The underlined words show how the meaning in the notes is presented in the patient's speech: they begin by describing their symptoms, and then they refer to the diagnosis. The word in bold must be the gap in the notes, as the back pain and numbness they experienced led to a diagnosis of sciatica.

Exercise

Take 20 seconds to look at the notes below, and underline the words that would help you to listen for the 3 gaps in the notes.

Treatment	• Began by taking orlistat and following the diet (limiting **(1)**_____, lots of vegetables)
	• After 6 months, began exercising gently, but found it difficult due to **(2)**_____.
	• After 12 months, no significant sustained weight loss.
	• Underwent **(3)**_____ in 2014 - no complications.

Exercise

Now, give yourself 20 seconds to look through the notes below, then answer questions 4 – 7.

Patient	Felix Leak
(A)	diagnosed with stage 1 testicular cancer in 2015
	underwent an orchidectomy in late 2015
	also given 2 cycles of chemotherapy following surgery
(B)	has recently experienced haematuria
	reports feeling tired, aching muscles
	describes the pain as 'always sore, but bearable'
(C)	works as an executive director at a law firm
	reports an increase in work-related stress following a recent promotion
	moderate drinker
	history of smoking

IMPROVE YOUR SCORE

Find a recording of a consultation online and listen and write down the:

a) names of symptoms

b) names of medications

c) names of tests/treatment options, etc.

(D)   book ultrasound scan

           give blood tests to check for tumour markers

4. For sections **(A)** – **(D)** of the text, describe the type of information being recorded.

5. How was the patient's cancer treated?

6. What is the most likely reason for Felix's recent consultation?

7. Where does Felix work?

Each consultation in Part A lasts for around 5 minutes, and usually covers the following areas of information.

1. Recent Medical History

Recent medical history is a common topic in Part A, as this section of the test is designed to test your ability to understand realistic patient language in English, and relating medical history is a common feature in consultations.

Exercise

Listen to **Track 1**, which gives an example of this section of a Part A consultation, and answer questions **8 – 11** below.

8.   How long ago did the patient's symptoms begin?

9.   What was the patient doing differently, as a result of the symptoms?

10.   In addition to being tired, what other symptoms did the patient have?

11.   What did Dr Lopez's blood tests show?

2. Other Medical History

You may also need to fill in gaps in the notes about the patient's more general medical history. This might include the patient's current medication, lifestyle choices, and past surgeries and illnesses.

Exercise

Take 10 seconds to scan the notes below, then play **Track 2**, and fill in blanks **12 – 15** as you listen.

IMPROVE YOUR SCORE

Use the 30 second pause before the recording plays to focus your listening. Underline words and phrases before and after the gaps in the notes, and listen for this information when the recording starts, so that you are prepared to listen for the answer.

Medical history	• **(12)** _____ throughout 2016 (no problems)
	• diagnosed with anaemia after feeling **(13)** _____ and tired
	• suffered from heavy periods
	• regularly **(14)** _____
	• broke arm and **(15)** _____ (2004)

3. Current Symptoms

In this section of the consultation, the health professional asks how the patient is currently feeling. Patients often describe their symptoms in everyday terms, using idioms and phrases that may be unfamiliar. It is your task to record what patients say about these issues. Not all the missing information will be medical terms – sometimes you will need to write down the word(s) the patient uses to describe the symptoms.

Exercise

 Take 10 seconds to scan the notes below, then play **Track 3**, and fill in blanks **16 – 19** as you listen.

Present Condition	• taking **(16)** _____ medication for the past 3 months
	• headaches in forehead, described as **(17)** _____
	• some nausea after food
	• hot flushes and sweating (clammy hands)
	• trouble sleeping, feeling **(18)** _____, and paranoid
	• former behaviours are reduced
	• is now **(19)** _____ about different things

IMPROVE YOUR SCORE

In the Listening Test, you hear speakers from a variety of English-speaking countries. You are likely to hear a range of accents on Test Day, including: American, Australian, Canadian, UK, Irish and New Zealand. These accents will be mild and easily understood. Search for podcasts and videos online created in these varieties of English to make sure you're familiar with the relevant accents, and are able to understand what these speakers are saying. The listening content in this book uses a range of speakers with various accents to help you to prepare.

4. Treatment

This section of the consultation discusses the patient's current and future treatment.
The patient may describe how they have been finding their treatment, or they may simply describe the treatment they have been following so far.

Exercise

 Take 10 seconds to scan the notes below, then play **Track 4** and fill in blanks **20 – 23** as you listen.

Treatment	• given **(20)** _____ by paramedics on way to hospital
	• morphine administered as pain relief
	• **(21)** _____ used under tongue to improve blood flow
	• observed **(22)** _____ using an EKG machine
	• **(23)** _____ procedure performed

In Part A of the Listening Test, you need to make sure you can keep up with the conversation and understand the key things that the speakers are saying. Familiarise yourself with common phrases and idioms in English, and practise listening to native English speakers use everyday language, to help you score well in this section on Test Day.

Listening Part A Practice Set

 Take 30 seconds to scan the patient notes on this page, then listen to **Track 5** and answer questions **1 – 12**.

Extract 1: Questions 1 to 12

You hear an optometrist talking to a new patient called Aidan Fitzpatrick. For **questions 1 to 12**, complete the notes with a word or short phrase.

Patient	Aidan Fitzpatrick
Symptoms	• first noticed difficulty reading two weeks ago
	• describes his vision as '**(1)** _____ ' ,
	• has difficulty reading printed letters
	• needs increasingly **(2)** _____ to read in evenings
	• found he was having to hold objects closer to see
	• purchased glasses from **(3)** _____
	• often finds that he's **(4)** _____ his eyes, even when wearing glasses
	• when struggling to see, can also experience **(5)** _____
	• Aidan treats pain with **(6)** _____ (fast-acting)
Background Details	• wore glasses as a child
	• brother also wears glasses, possibly **(7)** _____
Medical History	• recently suffered from **(8)** _____
	– treated with antibiotics
	– still experiencing symptoms of **(9)** _____
	• lost excess weight following a **(10)** _____ (describes as 'wakeup call')
Next Steps	• isn't willing to wear **(11)** _____
	• must be given **(12)** _____ (never had one)

IMPROVE YOUR SCORE

Part A is designed to test your ability to listen effectively to patients. As such, the gaps you need to fill in in Part A are generally found in the patient's speech. Make sure to pay attention to what the patient says about their treatment so far, their medical history, and their current symptoms.

Take 30 seconds to read through the patient notes on this page, then listen to
Track 6 and answer questions **13 – 24**.

Extract 1: Questions 13 to 24

You hear an obstetrician talking to a new patient called Hilary Johnson. For **questions 13 to
24**, complete the notes with a word or short phrase.

Patient	Hilary Johnson
Reason for referral	• glucose in **(13)** _____ indicates risk of diabetes
	• describes herself as **(14)** _____ sugary foods
	• noticed extra **(15)** _____ which may be unrelated to pregnancy
Family history of diabetes	• her **(16)** _____ suffers from diabetes (Type 2, controlled through diet)
Pregnancy symptoms	• morning sickness – pain in her **(17)** _____ , but no vomiting
	• **(18)** _____ controlled with medication
	• recently suffering from backache, described as '**(19)** _____' pain
	• has been feeling increasingly **(20)** _____
	• problems sleeping
	• concerned about diet (taking a **(21)** _____)
Occupation	• Secondary school teacher
	• feeling **(22)** _____, increased workload
Next appointment	• will take an **(23)** _____ glucose test (she's familiar with the procedure, a friend's had the test).
	• has been given a **(24)** _____ to consult ahead of her blood test

Answers

1	diet, limiting (*you would expect to listen for a type of food the patient no longer eats regularly*)
2	exercising, difficult due to (*you would expect to listen for something that makes exercising hard*)
3	underwent, 2014 (*you would expect to listen for a procedure the patient had in 2014*)
4	**(A)** medical history
	(B) current symptoms
	(C) lifestyle **OR** personal details
	(D) next steps **OR** treatment plan
5	orchidectomy
6	haematuria, tired, aching muscles
7	a law firm
8	2 months
9	going straight to bed
10	gaining weight, trouble focusing and paying attention
11	thyroxine was low
12	pregnant
13	dizzy
14	donated blood
15	(a couple of) ribs
16	fluoxetine
17	shooting pain
18	anxious
19	compulsive **OR** OCD
20	aspirin
21	nitro-glycerine
22	heart rhythms
23	angioplasty

Practice Sets

Questions 1 to 12

1	fuzzy
2	more light
3	(the) pharmacy
4	squinting
5	(a pretty persistent) headache
6	ibuprofen
7	short-sighted
8	sinusitis
9	(a) cold
10	myocardial infarction, or MI
11	contact lenses
12	(an) eye test

Questions 13 to 24

13	urine sample
14	craving
15	weight
16	aunt
17	stomach
18	heartburn
19	throbbing
20	tired
21	prenatal
22	(a little bit) stressed
23	oral
24	leaflet

Listening Transcripts

Track 1

F: Could you tell me, in your own words, what's brought you here today?

M: Yes, of course. Well, I went to see my general doctor, Dr Lopez, because I'd been feeling really tired. It had been going on for about two months, though I hadn't been to him sooner because I wasn't sure it was serious enough to warrant a visit to the doctor's – I'm generally the sort of person that just gets on with things, you know, I tend to let my body heal itself – but it got to the point where I was going straight to bed when I got home from my job, and not waking up until the morning. And I'd still be tired the next day, despite all that sleep! I also found that I was gaining weight, eating the same amount of food I've always had – maybe even less. I became a bit of a zombie, really. I had trouble focusing at work, and paying attention to what people were saying. It was my wife that eventually got me to go and see the doctor about it, she said I looked like I was on autopilot. Anyway, when I saw Dr Lopez he gave me lots of blood tests to see if I was lacking in anything… most everything turned out fine, but the blood tests showed that my… I think it was my thyroxine levels… were on the low side, so Dr Lopez referred me to you.

Track 2

F: Well, other than this, I'm not sure I've ever had any serious health problems. I suppose I had to visit the doctor a fair amount in 2016, because I was pregnant with my daughter… even that was fairly straightforward, there were no complications or concerns… then, I suppose a little while before that, I suffered from anaemia… I felt really tired, and I had dizzy spells. There were a bunch of different things that the doctors thought might be contributing to it: I was having heavy periods, and I donated blood as often as they'd let me… I think they also mentioned that caffeine could be an issue. I remember thinking it was weird that I had it, because at the time I was eating quite a lot of red meat, and I thought that was supposed to give you plenty of iron. Anyway, as soon as I visited the doctors they sorted me out… Other than that, I suppose the only health issue I can think of is falling off a bike in 2004 and breaking my arm. I broke a couple of ribs, as well, but they tend to sort themselves out. I had to wear a sling for a long time, with that arm. Sometimes it aches slightly; it's barely noticeable, though, and it might not be related.

Track 3

M: I just don't think that medication is doing me any good. For three months, ever since I started taking fluoxetine, I've been feeling really bizarre… I get these terrible headaches that come and go - it's like a shooting pain in my forehead - and I sometimes feel nauseous after eating… And I keep having these hot flushes, my hands will get clammy, and I feel anxious and start shaking! I find it difficult to sleep… umm when I'm in bed, I get kind of agitated, and I'll start thinking about all of the things that went wrong at work, or things that colleagues said to me… well, perhaps I feel a bit paranoid, I don't know. I just think it's really not worth all these side effects. I suppose I engage in my former OCD behaviour less, as a result of the medication? But I think that might just be because I'm spending my time worrying about everything else! It's like I've just swapped my former habits for new ones... I'm compulsive about different things now, like stressing at night. At least before, my OCD was only impacting parts of my day... these drugs, though! They're making my life so much more difficult.

Track 4

F: Okay, Mark, so can you tell me about what happened when you had your heart attack?

M: Yeah sure... It all happened really quickly, but I remember feeling this really weird chest pain, like a tightness in my chest, I told my wife my chest was hurting, and when I mentioned I had pains in my left arm she called an ambulance immediately... good thing she knew! So I remember the paramedics put me into the ambulance and gave me some aspirin. They took me to the ER and there they gave me a morphine shot for the pain I was feeling... umm... they also put a mask on me for oxygen to help me breath, and something under the tongue to help... I think it was to help my heart get more blood. It was called nitroglycerin. My wife was with me, I remember, and she was really great, really helped me to keep calm, although she told me later that she was freaking out! Then they hooked me up to an Electrocardiogram (ECG) machine to look at my heart rhythms. Evidently it must have showed some kind of blockage because they took me to the catheter lab straight away! I had to be operated on, they called it an angioplasty, because I was having a heart attack. The way they described it to me, it was basically like cleaning out the pipes that pumped blood to my heart muscle. They said that if I'd waited any longer to call an ambulance, the heart muscle would most likely have died from the lack of oxygen!

Track 5

N: You hear an optometrist talking to a patient called Aidan Fitzpatrick, who has been experiencing blurred vision.

F: Hi Aidan. I'm Dr Salkeld... could you start by telling me about what's been going on with your vision?

M: Sure... Well, I guess it must've started a while ago, but I didn't really notice it properly until about 2 weeks ago. I was working in my garden and I noticed that I was having a hard time reading the instructions on the gardening products that I'd just bought. I normally stick to the one I've been using for years, but I thought it'd be nice to try something different. Anyways, it kind of felt like everything was fuzzy around the edges, and I just couldn't see the letters clearly. After talking to my daughter, she mentioned that I'd been using increasingly more light to read at night and even pulling things closer to me to read. I hadn't even noticed! So I went out and got some of those glasses they sell at the pharmacy and they helped, but my doctor said that it'd be better if I came to see an eye doctor... Well they made things less blurred, anyway, I guess. My vision's still not crystal clear or anything when I use the glasses, but I wasn't really expecting that. I still notice that I'm squinting to see things... it's mostly when I'm trying to read something close-up, like small writing. I'm better when things are at a distance... I don't know if it's related – but I've also noticed a pretty persistent headache… I guess It's kind of at the sides of my head, I suppose. It comes and goes, but it's definitely worst when I'm having trouble seeing something. When it gets really bad, I just take a fast-acting ibuprofen, and that tends to sort it out.

F: Ever had any vision problems before?

M: When I was little, at some point in elementary school, I think I had glasses, but I'm sure I broke them and we just never got round to having them replaced. My brother has glasses that he's been wearing for years, I don't really know a whole lot about what's wrong with his eyes….maybe he's shortsighted? But that reminds me, my brother thought I should mention that a couple of months or so ago I was really pretty ill, I was suffering from sinusitis. And, anyway, I left it pretty late to go and see the doctor about it. Kind of thought that it would just sort itself out, anyway, it lingered for a while, so when I told my doctor he gave me some antibiotics and it cleared up pretty quickly after that. Well, for the most part… although I still feel like I have a cold. Other than that I've been in really good health for the last few years. I take my health really seriously, I'm not sure If the doctor told you, but I used to be quite overweight, but I lost it all after a bit of a wakeup call some years back… I had what you guys call a myocardial infraction… it was pretty scary, and I was quite overweight at the time, and really stressed out about my job. Since then I've made a real effort to look after myself properly.

F: I'm glad to hear it. So, in terms of your blurred vision, what do you think might work for you?

M: Well, I don't particularly like the idea of wearing glasses all the time, but touching my eyes freaks me out so contact lenses are definitely not an option. I guess the best thing might be to just have glasses that I wear all the time so I don't keep forgetting to put them on when I am out somewhere and not at home. I've actually never had an eye test, so I should probably schedule one of those as a next step.

F: I think that sounds reasonable. Let's do some tests to check out your eyes and go from there.

Track 6

M: Hilary Johnson? Hi, do come in and take a seat. I'm Dr Smith and I'm a senior obstetrician here… So, Hilary, you've been referred to us by your midwife. I have her notes with me here, but could you tell me in your own words why you've been referred?

F: Yeah, no problem… umm, I think I've been referred to you because the midwife said she found some glucose in my urine sample and was worried about diabetes. If I understand correctly, I could have diabetes during my pregnancy, but if I do, it's not likely to continue after giving birth? I've noticed that I'm craving sweets and cakes all the time at the moment, and I've just been letting myself eat whatever, so I've put on a bit of weight, and I don't think it's all just baby weight, either… I've never had a problem with diabetes before, and I'm hoping it will turn out to be something else. My aunt actually has type two diabetes, but she's always eaten a lot of sugar, so I think that might be a factor. She just controls hers with diet now and doesn't have to take any medication.

M: Oh. okay. Thanks for letting me know… I see from your notes that you're 24 weeks pregnant now, how has your pregnancy been up to now?

F: Oh, I've been so lucky! I got the usual sickness early on – well, you know, stomach pain, but not actually being sick – I think that's pretty common, and it settled after the first trimester. I've been taking some medication because I also had pretty horrible heartburn, and it seems to take care of the problem… and also I've started to get a bit of back pain in the last week or so… I'd say it's like a throbbing feeling but other than that I've been pretty fortunate. I suppose I've been gradually getting more and more tired since the start of my pregnancy. I've just put it down to the extra energy my baby needs, but it could also be because I haven't been sleeping very well. Also, sometimes the nausea stops me from making something healthy for dinner, which is annoying because I know I need to eat healthily. I take a prenatal, though, to make sure I'm getting the right nutrition.

M: Well, it seems like you're managing to deal with most of your symptoms well.

F: Yeah, this is my first pregnancy and to be honest I didn't have a clue what to expect but so far so good. It's only this glucose thing that's got me worried, I imagine it's just a one off but I guess it's best to get it seen to.

M: Certainly, and I'm pleased you're here so that we can get things sorted. So, we'll need to book another appointment to carry out some tests.

F: Okay, so when will I have to have this because, I'm a bit busy at work at the minute?

M: Well ideally as soon as possible. Can I ask what you do for a living?

F: I'm a high school teacher and it's just getting to that time of year where the kids are gearing up for their examinations. So I can't afford to be taking too much time off during the day. I'm actually a little bit stressed at the moment as well, I've had to do a lot more work over the past few weeks… I think it's just that time of year. I've been a teacher for 4 years now so I'm starting to develop ways of coping with the madness. With that in mind, if our next appointment could be at five-ish or later, then that would be perfect.

M: No problem, just make sure to let the receptionist know your preferences. When we find sugar in preliminary tests we offer an oral glucose tolerance test, which is what we'll do when you come in next. Do you know what that involves?

F: Well, I asked a few of my friends about their pregnancies and my friend Beth said that she had the same thing and told me about that test. She said that she had to come into the hospital and drink a sugary drink and then have a blood test to tell if she had diabetes. Is that right?

M: Yes that's pretty much it. Here is a leaflet that explains the test so that you can have a read about it when you get home. Do you have any other questions for me?

F: No I don't think so, I'll go away and read this, and wait and see what the test says. Thank you for your help today.

M: You're welcome. I'll see you once we have the results and we can take it from there.

Listening Part B

Introduction

In Part B of the Listening Test, you listen to 6 different short recordings in a healthcare setting and answer one question about each recording. Listening Part B tests your ability to understand and identify:

- the gist of the recording
- specific details within interactions
- the speaker's purpose
- the opinion of the speaker
- the actions that will result from the workplace communication.

Each of the 6 short listening tasks in Part B lasts for around 45 seconds, and the recording is heard only once. The recording will cover a workplace interaction involving healthcare professionals, such as a briefing or handover. You have 15 seconds to look at the question before each individual recording and 5 seconds to mark the answer after hearing the workplace communication

IMPROVE YOUR SCORE

There is only one question for each recording in Part B. Use the 15 second pause before the audio begins to focus on the question being asked, and think about how this question could be answered.

Strategies

Know the Instructions

You should make sure you are familiar with what you are asked to do before you take the test. The instructions look like this:

> In Part B of the Listening Test, you'll hear six different extracts. In each extract, you'll hear people talking in a different healthcare setting.

> For questions 25 to 30, choose the answer A, B or C which fits best according to what you hear.

Know the Context

Part B of the Listening Test contains 6 different recordings, each from a different healthcare setting. The recordings in this part of the test should be familiar to a healthcare professional from any of the 12 sectors covered by OET, because Part B tasks have generic, hospital-based contexts.

The recordings you hear in this section will contain one or two speakers. There is always at least one healthcare professional in each recording, and each recording will give an example of an everyday workplace interaction in a range of contexts.

Prepare for the Different Question Types

Use the 15 seconds before the recording begins to analyse the question. Don't look at any of the following questions during this time period, just focus on the question for the recording you are about to hear. When you look at the question, underline words that will help you to listen for the answer.

There are 7 different question types in Listening Part B: Gist, Detail, Speaker Purpose, Function, Opinion, Agreement and Future Actions.

1. Gist

Gist questions ask you to choose the option that correctly summarises the information heard in the recording. To answer these questions, you need to identify the idea, or gist, of the interaction. This question is looking for an overview of the information given in the audio, not a specific detail. The answer choices will report the information in the recording without repeating the exact words. This is the most common question type in the Part B section of the Listening Test. The following list gives examples of Gist questions:

> *What are the nurses talking about?*
> *The aim of the research was*
> *The vet is explaining that*

Exercise

 Play **Track 7** and answer questions **1** and **2**.

1. You hear a dentist discussing booking problems with her receptionist.

   What has caused the problem?

   Ⓐ an error with the booking system

   Ⓑ a double booked appointment

   Ⓒ a lack of communication

2. You hear a doctor discussing chest X-ray information with a medical student.

   What is the doctor explaining?

   Ⓐ the order for discussing results to the patient

   Ⓑ the information to include in patient notes

   Ⓒ how to correctly examine the patient's condition

2. Detail

Detail questions ask about a specific part of the recording. The detail asked for is often one of the central ideas in the recording, rather than a more trivial piece of information. You hear the information that allows you to answer the question – but the question may or may not use the actual words heard in the recording. The following list gives examples of Detail questions:

> *What would have improved the trainee's performance?*
>
> *The patient's medication has changed because*
>
> *What strategy does the surgeon suggest?*

Exercise

 Play **Track 8** and answer questions **3** and **4**.

3. You hear an ENT surgeon talking to a colleague about cochlear implants.

   The surgeon is explaining that cochlear implants

   Ⓐ transmit voices more clearly than other noises.

   Ⓑ emit a variety of sounds into a microphone.

   Ⓒ restore hearing in deaf people.

4. You hear a GP talk about diagnosing Type 2 diabetes mellitus.

   Why should a fasting plasma glucose test be booked in the morning?

   Ⓐ The patient will need to attend an 8 hour appointment.

   Ⓑ The test will need to be carried out twice.

   Ⓒ To allow the patient to eat during the day.

3. Speaker Purpose

Speaker Purpose questions ask about what one of the speakers is doing, or trying to do. To answer these questions, you need to understand why the speaker is saying what they are saying, and what result the speaker is aiming for. The following list gives examples of Speaker Purpose questions:

> *What does he want to know about his treatment?*
>
> *The doctor explains that the practice should*
>
> *The trainee is trying to understand*

Exercise

 Play **Track 9** and answer questions **5** and **6**.

5. You hear a dentist talking to a patient with a chipped tooth.

    What does the patient want to know?

    (A) how long the procedure will last

    (B) when her next appointment will be

    (C) what her different treatment options are

6. You hear a podiatrist talking to a patient with fallen arches

    The patient explains that his treatment

    (A) will need to continue for some time.

    (B) has become too time-consuming.

    (C) is not improving his condition.

4. Function

Function questions ask about what one of the speakers is doing, or what the function of what they are saying is. To answer these questions correctly, you need to understand the actions that their language describes. The following list gives examples of Function questions:

> *What is the dentist doing?*
>
> *Why has the patient called the doctor?*

Exercise

 Play **Track 10** and answer questions **7** and **8**.

7. You hear a doctor talking to a patient in an emergency department.

    What is the doctor doing?

    (A) explaining how the patient will be treated

    (B) reassuring the patient that she is not at risk

    (C) going over the cause of the patient's infection

8. You hear a medical student talking to a senior resident about assessing a patient.

    What is the senior resident doing?

    (A) teaching the student how to examine the patient

    (B) explaining when to prescribe additional medications

    (C) showing the student where to observe the jugular vein

5. Opinion

Opinion questions ask you to identify the opinion of a speaker on the issue discussed. When answering Opinion questions, pay attention to how the speakers say things, and their attitude towards the topic in the question. The following list gives examples of Opinion questions:

> *The radiographer thinks that the patient*
>
> *How does she feel about her role?*
>
> *The nurse believes that the doctor*

Exercise

   Play **Track 11** and answer question **9**.

9. You hear a psychiatrist presenting a case study.

    What did the psychiatrist find unusual about the case?

    (A) The symptoms suggested a different cause.

    (B) Effects were experienced long after the cause.

    (C) The cause of the illness could not be determined.

6. Agreement

Agreement questions ask you to identify what the speakers are in agreement about. To answer these questions correctly, listen to the conversation and pay attention to the reactions of each speaker to the other's suggestions .The following list gives examples of Agreement questions:

> *The speech pathologist agrees that*
>
> *What do they agree about?*
>
> *The physiotherapists agree that they will*

Exercise

   Play **Track 12** and answer question **10**.

10. You hear a dietitian talking with a patient.

    What do they agree about?

    (A) The patient has forgotten their overall goal.

    (B) The patient has been too severe with their diet.

    (C) The patient has been trying to lose too much weight.

7. Course of Action

Course of Action questions ask you to decide what the speakers will do as a result of the conversation or talk. Pay attention to anything that will be done later while listening to the recording, and be aware of when in the future the actions will be done. For example, a speaker may talk about what needs to be done tonight, and what should be done tomorrow. The question specifies which of these actions is correct. The following list gives examples of Course of Action questions:

What does the nurse have to do next?

What will the doctor do tonight?

Next week, the patient must

Exercise

 Play **Track 13** and answer question **11**.

11. You hear a veterinarian talking with an owner.

   What will the owner do later today?

   (A) give his cat plenty of attention

   (B) give his cat drugs to reduce overgrooming

   (C) give his cat food at the same time as last night

On Test Day, you should aim to identify the focus of the question during your 15 seconds of scanning time before the audio begins, so that you know the type of information to listen for in the audio. Once you have identified the question type, you should look for important words in the question, and think of paraphrases for the answer choices. Then, when the audio starts, you will be prepared to listen for the right information.

IMPROVE YOUR SCORE

Many Part B recordings are between two healthcare professionals in a workplace setting, and they can also include patients. You might find it helpful to watch a television programme set in a hospital from the UK, Australia, the US, or another English speaking country. While these programmes will rarely discuss healthcare in a technical way, they will help you familiarise yourself with common vocabulary and interactions in an English speaking healthcare setting.

Listening Part B Practice Set

For questions **1 to 6**, choose the answer A, B or C which fits best according to what you hear.

 Play **Track 14** and answer questions **1 – 6**.

1. You hear an ED nurse talking to the relative of a patient who has been recently admitted.

    What is the relative doing?

    (A) describing her father's medical history

    (B) suggesting ways to interact with her father

    (C) explaining that her father can become violent

2. You hear an obstetrician describing a caesarean section to a pregnant patient.

    He says that the procedure will

    (A) be shorter and less painful than a traditional birth.

    (B) be carried out while the patient is conscious.

    (C) not be necessary in the patient's case.

3. You hear a GP and his practice nurse discussing their yearly schedule.

    They agree that the practice should

    (A) hire agency staff to help during the busier weeks.

    (B) avoid taking holiday in the beginning of September.

    (C) look after their health, to lower the likelihood of sickness.

4. You hear a nurse preparing a patient for a flu shot.

    What is the nurse doing?

    (A) explaining why the flu shot is necessary

    (B) discussing why the flu shot causes reactions

    (C) describing common side effects of the flu shot

5. You hear a doctor talking to a patient about her injury.

    What will happen when the patient returns to the surgery?

    (A) She will have her stitches removed.

    (B) The doctor will stitch up her wound.

    (C) They will see if the wound will scar.

6. You hear a trainee nurse asking a senior colleague about the treatment for a patient with chronic obstructive pulmonary disease, or COPD.

    The senior colleague is explaining that giving such patients normal levels of oxygen

    (A) can inhibit breathing rate.

    (B) will cause light-headedness.

    (C) lowers carbon dioxide levels.

Answers

1	C	a lack of communication.
2	B	The information to include in patient notes.
3	A	transmit voices more clearly than other noises.
4	C	To allow the patient to eat during the day.
5	C	what her different treatment options are
6	C	is not improving his condition.
7	A	explaining how the patient will be treated
8	A	teaching the student how to examine the patient
9	B	Effects were experienced long after the cause.
10	B	The patient has been too severe with their diet.
11	A	give his cat plenty of attention

Practice Set

1	C	explaining that her father can become violent
2	B	be carried out while the patient is conscious.
3	B	avoid taking holiday in the beginning of September.
4	C	describing common side effects of the flu shot
5	A	She will have her stitches removed.
6	A	can inhibit breathing rate.

Listening Transcripts

Track 7

N: You hear a dentist discussing booking problems with her receptionist.

F: Hey Kieran, Mr Lao just mentioned that he'd tried to reschedule his appointment yesterday, first online, and then, when that didn't work, he called up. But apparently he couldn't reschedule... any idea why?

M: Hmm... I wasn't working yesterday, but let me check the notes... so, Lana left a note about the call. She says that Mr Lao wanted to reschedule, but we didn't have any other appointments this week after 3 pm, which is the only time he could make. He asked if he could make an appointment next week, but his procedure was marked on our system as 'urgent', so she had to make it in the same week – the system wouldn't have let her reschedule it any later. She wouldn't have had the authorisation to change that ... still, she should have discussed this with you at lunch or at the end of the day, because then you could have decided whether it could have been postponed for a week.

F: Yeah... In his circumstance, it would have been fine to reschedule at a slightly later date. We should prevent something like this from happening again.

M: Mmm, you're right. I'll talk to her about it tomorrow, and I'll send out an email to everyone else, so that they're aware.

N: You hear a doctor discussing chest X-ray information with a medical student.

F: Hey, Dr Yan, we've got the X-rays back for Mr Regis in bed eight... from this morning.

M: Great, can you document them in the notes?

F: Umm... Do you mind showing me how to write the interpretation properly?

M: Of course. Make sure you put the patient details: full name, date of birth, patient number and home address first. Then put the hospital and ward, date and time. Make sure your name is on the document, too. Include the indication for the X-ray like "haemoptysis" or "dyspnea" before documenting your interpretation. Now, I use a simple mnemonic to make sure I don't miss anything, ABCDE: Airway – trachea, carina, bronchi and the hilar structures; Breathing – lung fields and pleura; Cardiac – heart size and heart borders; Diaphragm – position, shape and costophrenic angles. Finally, Everything else: the mediastinal contours, bones and tubes or devices. Make sure you document everything clearly using this system in the notes.

Track 8

N: You hear an ENT surgeon talking to a colleague about cochlear implants.

M: We implant an electrode array, which looks like several small wires made of a platinum-iridium alloy into different regions of the cochlea. These metal wires conduct the electrical impulses generated from the microphone, which picks up sound from the environment and sends the signals to the electrode array through a transmitter. There's also a speech processor between the two that filters more important sounds so that the patient can hear people talking rather than other sounds.

F: Right, okay. So does this restore hearing to normal levels?

M: No, with the current technology, we're giving deaf people a good representation of sounds from the environment and help to understand speech. After surgery, patients undergo therapy to relearn their sense of hearing. Not everyone benefits from the device to the same extent.

N: You hear a GP talk about Type 2 diabetes mellitus.

F: Hello! I'll be covering the diagnosis of Type 2 diabetes mellitus. So, there are four methods that we can use. The first is a fasting plasma glucose test. This is our preferred diagnostic test, as it's easier to carry-out, often more convenient, and costs us less than the other three tests. It helps to try and book these appointments in the morning, as the patient has to refrain from eating for at least eight hours before they can take the test. Normal fasting blood glucose will be between 70 and 100 milligrams per deciliter. A value of over 126 milligrams per deciliter indicates a diagnosis of diabetes. Bear in mind that this test should be carried out twice to confirm a positive result. The second method we can use is to measure the average glycemic load over the past three months...

Track 9

N: You hear a dentist talking to a patient with a chipped tooth.

M: So we've talked about different options, and it seems like a veneer would be the best treatment. Given the cost of the procedure, are you happy to go ahead?

F: It's quite expensive, but I definitely need to get it fixed. Will it stay put?

M: Veneers tend to need replacing every ten to fifteen years, so they are a long-term solution. It will certainly be more durable than composite bonding, and it will look more realistic, too.

F: Ah, okay that's great. And is there anything I can do to extend their lifespan?

M: Well, you need to maintain good oral health, you know, brushing, flossing, regular check-ups. You should avoid brushing your veneer too hard, as it could cause damage.

N: You hear a podiatrist talking to a patient with fallen arches.

F: So you say you're experiencing foot pain, are you wearing supportive shoes?

M: Uh-hu, I'm wearing appropriate shoes, and I'm also wearing orthotics that should be helping, but I'm still experiencing pain in my feet. Sometimes they feel a bit numb, too.

F: Right, okay. And you mentioned that you've been given some foot exercises to do?

M: Yeah, the physiotherapist I went to showed me those. At first I thought they were helping, but now I think I'm as bad as I've ever been. Is there anything else we can do?

Track 10

N: You hear a doctor talking to a patient in an emergency department.

M: Hello again, I'm Dr Oliveira, I think we met earlier at the beginning of my shift. How are you doing now, Mrs James?

F: I don't really know what's going on, I'm just hoping to find out what's wrong with me.

M: Okay Mrs James, I understand, and thank you for waiting. They've run the tests and they think you've got a condition called pseudomembranous colitis. It's a long way of saying you've got an inflamed colon. You've been waiting so long here in A&E because you're going to need a side room, because of the infection risk.

F: Oh dear, thank you for telling me. How long will it be till I get a room? Is it serious?

M: Well, at the moment, Mrs James, we're operating on a 'one in, one out basis'... but I do think that a side room will free up in the next few hours. The outlook is very good in most cases, we're going to give you antibiotics and fluids but there is a small risk of the infection returning in the future.

N: You hear a medical student talking to a senior resident about assessing a patient.

M: I understand that Mr Fredrick has chronic heart failure, and that we are concerned with volume overload if he doesn't adequately excrete enough fluid. But how do we determine his volume status and whether or not he needs diuretic medications?

F: That is a good question! So, there are several ways we can assess volume status. First, we can perform a physical examination on the patient. What would we be looking for?

M: Well, we can assess for peripheral edema. We would look at the patients hands and feet to assess swelling and determine whether or not there is pitting.

F: Yes! Very good. We can also assess for jugular venous pressure. This is most easily done by having the patient lay at a 45 degree incline and then observing his external jugular vein. The filling level of the jugular vein should be less than 3 centimetres above the sternal angle.

Track 11

N: You hear a psychiatrist presenting a case study.

M: Good morning everyone! I would like to speak about a curious case that I was involved in last year. The patient was a young man who reported continued visual disturbances.

What made this case so interesting were the changes he described to his visual field. Objects began to get larger and smaller as he looked at them, his father's face slowly morphed into that of a stranger, and he would see trails of light zigzagging across his field of view. These are uncommon for visual hallucinations, they are unlikely characteristics of a primary psychotic disorder, but they *are* akin to a psychoactive substance-induced hallucination. However, his urine drug screen was negative for any substances, and he reported that his last use of any hallucinogen was three months ago! We have found several case reports of Hallucinogen Persisting Perception Disorder (HPPD) and believe that this patient matches the criteria for such a diagnosis.

Track 12

N: You hear a dietician talking with a patient.

F: Okay, Mr Weiss, so it looks like you haven't lost any weight this month… Do you have any idea why that might be?

M: Ugh… really? I feel like I've been trying really hard to lose weight. In fact, I thought I would take it a step further in the past couple of weeks, because I was a bit bad in the first week or so. So recently I've been trying to cut out all carbs, and any junk food. To be completely honest though… I've wound up cheating on my diet.

F: You need to stop being so strict with yourself. We designed your diet so that it would be achievable. When you try and do things too quickly, and make too many changes to what your body is used to, it's difficult to maintain long-term, and you end up overeating as a result. Also, I can't imagine that it made you feel good about your progress, when you kept going off track?

M: No, it really didn't. I see what you're saying… I guess I need to be kinder to myself, and be more patient with the slow and steady route.

Track 13

N: You hear a vet discussing treatment with a cat's owner.

F: Yeah… I've seen this before. Typically, when cats bite their fur off, or overgroom themselves, it's a sign of anxiety. Can you think of anything that might be causing Felix to become stressed?

M: Urrr… gosh, that makes me feel terrible! Well, I suppose we have moved house recently, and I've tried to get Felix to explore our back yard, but the neighbours have a dog that barks, and I guess that's been scaring him. Also, I've been working late quite often, so I suppose he's getting fed later than usual, and seeing me less. But there's really nothing I can do at the moment, I have a deadline that I have to meet this week, so I'll be working late until then.

F: Right, okay… In that case, I'd suggest trying to implement a couple of changes at home, starting next week. You should set a regular time for Felix's dinner, and stick to it. If you have to work late, can you arrange for Felix to be fed by someone else? Also, and you should start this as soon as you get home, you need to make sure you're spending enough time with Felix every day. If he isn't going out, then you're the only person he'll see each day. I'll schedule another appointment in a month to review, if he's still overgrooming his back, we can put him on a course of medication, to help with anxiety.

Track 14

N: You hear an ED nurse talking to the relative of a patient who has been recently admitted.

M: Did you want to talk to me, Miss Tanaka?

F: Oh… yes, you see, I just wanted to let you know that my father… well, as you know, he's recently been diagnosed with dementia… most of the time it's not an issue, and his spats never last long. It's just that I wanted to prepare you, sometimes he's really not himself.

M: Ah, okay, Miss Tanaka, I think I understand. Can your father become aggressive?

F: Yes… I mean, I think it's just that he gets frustrated sometimes. He can't remember things, and I think it's scary for him. He was never, ever like this before his dementia, and those periods, well, they really don't reflect his true character.

M: Of course, thanks for letting me know.

N: You hear an obstetrician describe a caesarean section to a pregnant patient.

M: Labour can progress differently for different people. In some circumstances, if labour is longer than expected and if we detect that the baby is distressed then we may have to consider an emergecy caesarean section. It's a procedure that we perform in theatre and it is carried out under spinal or epidural anaesthetic, so that you don't feel anything, but you will be awake. A screen is placed across your body so you don't have to see what's being done. We make an incision in your tummy and womb, just under your bikini line, to remove your baby and then stitch up the wound. It takes around 40 minutes and your birth partner can be there at all times. Does that make sense?

N: You hear a GP and his practice nurse discussing their yearly schedule.

M: In September we'll have a lot of new patients, as the first year university students will all register during freshers.

F: Yes, we were really run off our feet last year, weren't we?

M: Yep. It was a mad house.

F: Do you think we should hire agency staff to help out for the first couple of weeks this time around?

M: Well, I think part of the problem was that last year, Dr Igwe and Nurse Fletcher were both away – Dr Igwe went to Costa Rica, and Nurse Fletcher had the flu.

F: Right! I remember. Well, we can't do much to prevent staff illness.

M: No, but we can ask people to avoid booking time off in those first three weeks.

F: Okay, I'll send an email out today.

N: You hear a nurse prepare a patient for a flu shot.

F: Good morning Mr. Henderson, Dr. Ray has recommended that you get a flu immunisation shot before you are discharged. I've got the injection ready to give to you. Are you allergic to anything?

M: I'm only allergic to latex and penicillin. I don't know if I want the flu shot. The last time I got the shot, I got sick.

F: I'm sorry that happened to you. What kind of symptoms did you have after that last flu shot?

M: I got a runny nose and a headache. My arm felt like someone punched me.

F: Sometimes the flu shot can cause reactions like a sore injection site and headache. Other common symptoms include being tired, muscle and joint aches, shivering and fever. All of these symptoms can be seen with the flu, but the shot can't give you the flu.

N: You hear a doctor talk to a patient about her injury.

M: Good morning, Mrs. Bowder. I'll be your doctor taking care of your cut there. What exactly happened?

F: It's embarrassing really, you see, I was just trying to chop some tomatoes for dinner and the knife accidentally slipped. Oh, I'm so clumsy, I hope it doesn't hurt too much to stitch back up!

M: Well, we're going to numb the area now with a shot of Lidocaine. You'll feel a poke of the needle and a slight burn, but afterwards the area should be numb and you'll feel nothing during the procedure. We should be finished in about 10 minutes.

F: Oh good! How many stitches will I need? How long will they have to stay in? I'm really conscious about my hands so I hope I don't have a scar.

M: I will only know for sure once I finish suturing, but by my estimation, you might require at least four to five sutures. They'll have to stay in for 5 to 10 days and you will need to come back in to get them removed. I'll do my best to try and line the edges up to create as little scarring as possible, but I can't guarantee there will be nothing there!

N: You hear a trainee nurse asking a senior colleague about the treatment for a patient with chronic obstructive pulmonary disease, or COPD.

M: I haven't treated anyone with COPD before; what would we need to do differently?

F: One of the most important things would be to make sure to prescribe oxygen at levels between 88 – 92%.

M: Okay... so why would that be necessary? If he's having trouble breathing, shouldn't we prescribe higher oxygen levels? Most patients receive oxygen at levels between 94 – 98%.

F: Well, in healthy individuals, a rise in carbon dioxide would result in an increased drive to breathe in order to eliminate the excess gas.

M: Right.

F: However, in some patients with COPD, this response is blunted and their main mechanism for respiratory drive is controlled by the level of oxygen in the body instead. If the level of oxygen given to a COPD patient is increased too much, it can actually reduce the stimulus to breathe and cause hypoventilation, resulting in an increase in CO2.

Listening Part C

Introduction

In Listening Part C, you need to listen to two recordings, which can be either presentations or interviews involving a healthcare professional, and answer 6 multiple-choice questions for each one. Each recording lasts around 4 – 5 minutes.

The recordings in this section could be in the form of a workplace presentation or podcast-style interview. There will be a range of topics of broad healthcare interest.

Strategies

Know the Instructions

You should make sure you are familiar with what you have to do before you take the test. The instructions look like this:

> In this part of the test, you'll hear two different extracts. In each extract, you'll hear health professionals talking about aspects of their work.
>
> For **questions 31 to 42**, choose the answer (**A**, **B** or **C**) which fits best according to what you hear.
>
> **Extract 1: Questions 31 to 36**
>
> You hear a Senior Nurse called Pierre Delacroix giving a presentation about adrenal fatigue.

The first part of these instructions is the same for the beginning of each Part C test; you hear a general introduction to Part C, then the context sentence and specific instructions for each task. In the example above, for example, you would expect to hear a workplace presentation.

In Listening Part C, you hear either a presentation or an interview in each recording. A presentation in Part C has only one speaker, who will talk about a number of different points. An interview in Part C includes 2 speakers; one is a healthcare expert, and the other is the interviewer. The interviewer asks short questions, and the healthcare expert gives long answers to these questions. The interviewer's questions always relate to the question you need to answer in the section you're listening to at that point.

Scan the Questions

Before the recording begins, you have 30 seconds to read through the questions. When looking at the questions, pay attention to the words in the question and the answer choices. The words in the question will help you to identify the relevant part of the recording, and the correct answer can be heard in the recording shortly after this. To select the correct answer, you will need to choose the option that best reflects the meaning of what you hear in the recording. The questions in Part C tend to ask for the general meaning, or gist, of the section of speech. These questions also aim to test your understanding of the arguments the speaker talks about, and the attitude or opinion of the speaker.

Listen Actively, and Answer the Questions

In Part C of the Listening Test, you have to keep track of which question the recording is referring to. You need to answer 6 questions while the recording continues, so it's important that you know when to move on to the next question. The recording includes cues that you can use to identify when to move onto the next question – for example, the interviewer's questions in a recording match the questions in the task, and a presentation will follow a similar structure, using words in the presentation to highlight which parts of the recording relate to which questions. Be sure to read the questions carefully before the recording begins so you have a clear idea of what the audio for each question covers – use this knowledge to keep you on track throughout this part of the test.

Look at the question and answer choices in the exercise below, and look for words in the text to listen out for before you play the recording.

IMPROVE YOUR SCORE

Don't worry if the speakers are talking about a topic you're not familiar with. The listening section of OET is designed to be understood by healthcare professionals from a variety of backgrounds, so even if the topic is unfamiliar to you, all the information needed to answer the questions is given in the recording.

Exercise

You hear a General Practitioner called Dr Jeffords giving a presentation about patient referrals.

 Take 5 seconds to look at the question, then listen to **Track 15** and answer question **1**.

1.   Why does Dr Jeffords think it's important to ask patients why they're taking certain medication?

    (A)   to understand their medical history

    (B)   to measure the patient's awareness

    (C)   to question its effectiveness

Listening to Interviews

When listening to an interview, use the interviewer's questions as cues to move on to the next question. Pay attention to the keywords in the questions, as these are often reflected in the question you need to answer. Practise answering the questions for each section and moving on to the following question in time by completing the exercise below.

Exercise

You hear an interview with a vet called Amanda Chen about feline immunodeficiency virus (FIV).

 Take 15 seconds to scan the questions, then listen to **Track 16** and answer questions **2 – 4**.

2.   Dr Chen explains that many people believe FIV

    (A)   can be contagious to humans.

    (B)   might affect their pet's behaviour.

    (C)   has minimal impact on a cat's life.

3.   What does Dr Chen say people find confusing about the virus?

    (A)   the lack of available information

    (B)   the many different treatment options

    (C)   its name is similar to a more serious illness

IMPROVE YOUR SCORE

Remember to read the questions first and underline any important words, so that you can listen actively for the answers when the speakers begin talking.

4. Dr Chen advises those who own FIV positive cats to

    (A) avoid unnecessary contact.

    (B) monitor the pet's health carefully.

    (C) ensure the pet receives enough exercise.

Listening to Results of Trials

Speakers in Listening Part C often mention research trials that they have undertaken, or that they are aware of, or surveys that have been completed, which are relevant to their research topic. You should be prepared to answer questions about trials and patient surveys during this part of the test.

Exercise

You hear a hospital doctor called Dr Abu Mohammed giving a presentation on the results of a recent patient survey.

 Take 10 seconds to scan the questions, then listen to **Track 17** and answer questions 5 – 6.

5. Dr Mohammed was surprised by the year-long survey on the satisfaction of patients staying in hospital because of the

    (A) happiness of the patients.

    (B) severity of most patients' conditions.

    (C) number of patients that got involved.

6. Why does Dr Mohammed suggest patients in their 20s were more satisfied than the rest of the patients surveyed in the study?

    (A) They were more optimistic.

    (B) They spent less time in hospital.

    (C) They showed a greater rate of recovery.

Case Studies

In Part C, health professionals often discuss case studies. Questions in this section focus on the individual patient's experiences, what was unusual about their treatment, and how effective the treatment was. Practise answering questions about specific patients by completing the exercise below.

Exercise

You hear a nurse called Jonathan McKenzie giving a presentation on treating patients who are dealing with stress.

 Take 10 seconds to scan the questions, then listen to **Track 18** and answer questions **7 – 8**.

7.   Nurse McKenzie says that the CEO had trouble managing stress because

   Ⓐ   it was prolonged.

   Ⓑ   it was causing him to lose hours of sleep.

   Ⓒ   he was unfamiliar with such situations.

8.   The patient was encouraged to read because

   Ⓐ   it was a hobby of his.

   Ⓑ   it created a relaxing atmosphere.

   Ⓒ   he needed to learn about the cause of his issues.

In Part C of the Listening Test, you must show that you are able to follow a healthcare professional talking in detail on a healthcare topic. Practise listening to podcasts and presentations online covering healthcare topics, and make notes on the topic as you listen.

Listening Part C Practice Set

Part C

In this part of the test, you'll hear two different extracts. In each extract, you'll hear health professionals talking about aspects of their work.

For **questions 1 to 12**, choose the answer (**A**, **B** or **C**) which fits best according to what you hear.

Extract 1: Questions 1 to 6

You hear an interview with Dr Tadita Hussein, who's talking about treating patients with cystic fibrosis.

 Take 30 seconds to scan the questions, then play **Track 19** and answer questions **1 – 6**.

1. Dr Hussein says that patients with cystic fibrosis

    (A) may find the side effects alarming.

    (B) tend to require treatment from a young age.

    (C) can improve their condition with frequent hospital visits.

2. What does Dr Hussain say is difficult when treating patients who are not in hospital?

    (A) They often find the exercises too complicated.

    (B) They tend to have difficulty socialising with other people.

    (C) They don't always understand the importance of their treatment.

3. What does Dr Hussein say about the role of 'distraction therapy' in cystic fibrosis treatment?

    (A) It can be related to the treatment being provided.

    (B) It allows patients to complete their activities more quickly.

    (C) It provides staff with more information about the patient's condition.

4. What changes did Dr Hussein observe in one of her patients?

    (A) He showed respiratory improvement.

    (B) He deteriorated rapidly following a change in treatment.

    (C) He began to enjoy aspects of their treatment.

5. Dr Hussein plans to use technology to help cystic fibrosis patients to communicate

     A with other patients who suffer from the condition.

     B with family members who cannot visit them in hospital.

     C with patients of a similar age suffering from different conditions.

6. Dr Hussein suggests that future treatments for cystic fibrosis

     A will always incorporate lengthy procedures.

     B could prevent breathing difficulties in sufferers.

     C might be less painful than the current options available.

Extract 2: Questions 7 to 12

You hear an presentation given by Dr Hubert Johnson, who's talking about ways to improve efficiency.

 Take 30 seconds to scan the questions, then play **Track 20** and answer questions 7 – 12.

7. Dr Johnson explains that delays are increased when patients believe

     A their appointment will not begin on time.

     B staff are not concerned about late-arrivals.

     C being late for appointments will not impact others.

8. Dr Johnson uses an example of poor efficiency to illustrate the point that

     A healthcare professionals should assist staff during busy times.

     B practices should avoid limiting appointment booking options.

     C staff should be trained to handle demanding situations.

9. Dr Johnson explains that, in order to improve efficiency, healthcare practices must

     A sanction patients arriving later than 10 minutes.

     B avoid booking appointments in the morning.

     C show patients that they can run on time.

10. Dr Johnson says healthcare professionals often forget that patients who book appointments must first

     A feel that they need a consultation.

     B find a time and date that works for them.

     C consider what might be causing their issue.

11. What happened when Dr Johnson began giving weekly presentations to patients?

    (A) Dr Johnson was able to work fewer hours.

    (B) The general health of patients was increased.

    (C) The number of appointments at the practice decreased.

12. How does Dr Johnson feel about the use of technology when booking appointments?

    (A) Practices should begin to encourage all patients to make bookings online.

    (B) It can increase efficiency if other booking methods are continued.

    (C) Elderly people are most likely to struggle to use it.

Answers

1	**B** to measure the patient's awareness
2	**A** can be contagious to humans.
3	**C** its name is similar to a more serious virus
4	**B** monitor their health carefully.
5	**C** amount of patients that got involved.
6	**B** They spent less time in hospital.
7	**A** the stressful situation was prolonged.
8	**A** it was a hobby of his.

Practice Sets

Questions 1 to 6

1	**B** tend to require treatment from a young age.
2	**C** They don't always understand the importance of their treatment.
3	**A** It can be related to the treatment being provided.
4	**C** He began to enjoy aspects of their treatment.
5	**C** He began to enjoy aspects of their treatment.
6	**B** could prevent breathing difficulties in sufferers.

Questions 7 to 12

7	**A** their appointment will not begin on time
8	**B** practices should avoid limiting appointment booking options.
9	**C** show patients that they can run on time.
10	**A** feel that they need a consultation.
11	**C** The number of appointments at the practice decreased.
12	**B** It can increase efficiency if other booking methods are continued.

Listening Transcripts

Track 15

M: When dealing with new patients or patient referrals, you need to ask not only what medication they're currently taking, but why they're taking it. Many doctors assume that patients understand the reasons for their course of treatment, but some patients may have been prescribed these drugs a long time ago, and despite their prior doctor no doubt outlining the reasons why such drugs are needed, patients can forget, or mis-remember the actual reason why these prescriptions are necessary to them. Make sure you go through this at the earliest convenience – so a good way to start these discussions is to ask 'Can you tell me what you're currently taking, and what it's for?'

Track 16

M: Today I'm talking to Dr Chen, a veterinary expert in feline immunodeficiency virus, or FIV. Dr. Chen, what can you tell us about the disease?

F: Well, FIV is a topic that I tend to discuss quite frequently with my patients. Although lots of people have heard of FIV, and know generally that it is a virus that affects cats, there are many misconceptions about the condition, what it means for the cat, and what owners with FIV positive cats must do. Many people worry about catching FIV from infected cats, which is actually not possible, as the disease cannot be transmitted to humans. Unfortunately, this belief often prevents people from adopting cats who suffer from FIV, as they're concerned about themselves or their children contracting the virus from the cat.

M: I see... and are there any other things that might confuse people about FIV?

F: There certainly are! There is another virus that can affect cats that people may be aware of, called Feline Leukemia, or FeLV. FeLV significantly reduces a cat's life expectancy and health. Due to the similarity of the two virus's names, I've found that people tend to mix the two viruses up, so when they're told that a cat has FIV, they believe that the cat is extremely ill, and will require lengthy and expensive treatment, when in fact, the cat should be able to lead a fairly normal life.

M: I'm sure many owners will be relieved to hear that! So, what advice would you give to owners of FIV positive cats?

F: Well, the virus can deplete certain white blood cells, which means that cats with FIV are often more susceptible to catching other infections, and will often find it more difficult to recover from these infections. FIV is often compared to AIDS in humans, and the two immunosuppressant viruses are very similar. Those with FIV positive cats should by and large treat their cats the same as any other cats. However, these cats should be kept indoors, to lower the risk of infection, and to prevent them from spreading the virus. Owners should also pay more attention to the well-being of their cat, and if their pet shows any sign of illness, they should be taken to the vet at the earliest opportunity.

Track 17

M: As healthcare workers, we always put our patients first. We've recently concluded a year-long survey, looking into the level of satisfaction of adult in-patients at this hospital, and I wanted to share some of those results with you all today. I've been doing these surveys for a while now, and let me tell you, first off, that I was absolutely flabbergasted by the patient engagement level here. Seriously, out of all of the patients asked to complete this survey, a remarkable 86% responded. That may be the highest proportion I've ever seen! More responses not only provide us with more data, but it also suggests that you've created a great environment in which your patients feel comfortable expressing their views.

Let's take a look at what some of these respondents felt about the care they received. We'll start with in-patients in their 20s. This group had the highest satisfaction rate of all respondents. Now, that's great, but there are a couple of influencing factors we should bear in mind, that might explain why this group was more satisfied with their treatment. The group of patients in their 20s was also the group with the shortest average in-patient stay. The majority of these patients were discharged after less than a week in hospital. As such, this group is less likely to have experienced the frustration and worry that can become more of an issue with patients who have extended stays at the hospital.

Track 18

M: Hi everyone. I'd like to talk to you all about caring for patients experiencing stress. Unfortunately, it's a phenomenon many of us healthcare professionals have first-hand experience with, but I'm going to talk about one of my patients, a newly appointed CEO of a well-known multinational company. Now, the patient had been working in high-powered roles for a long time, so it wasn't that he was unfamiliar with stress. The problem was that in his current role, he was constantly putting out fires. The business was very well-known, and dominated the market that it was in, but behind the scenes there were financial issues. There was always an issue that needed his urgent attention. Stress is an unpleasant experience in and of itself, but it can also cause problematic side effects. The patient also experienced weight gain, and trouble sleeping as a result.

The patient waited for a while before seeking help, and by the time he did, he was absolutely worn out. We worked with the patient to develop a number of coping strategies, as it wasn't possible for him to remove the main cause of stress – his job – from his life. Instead, our treatment began with reading. The patient told us that he had loved reading fiction, but hadn't read for pleasure in decades, and so one of the first changes he made was to read for an hour before bed. We needed to make sure the patient made time for activities that he enjoyed. That one small change, in turn, helped him to sleep better, which gave him more energy to deal with stressful situations during the day.

Track 19

M: Cystic fibrosis is a condition that causes mucus to be thicker and stickier than it should be. Dr Tadita Hussein specialises in cystic fibrosis treatment, and is here to share her thoughts on caring for people with the condition. Tadita, can you tell us a bit more about patients who suffer from cystic fibrosis?

F: Absolutely. Sufferers tend to carry two to five times as much salt in their bodies as those without the condition, so you can see why their mucus is thicker than average. Treatment for these patients is usually quite time consuming and repetitive, patients are often required to stay in hospital for long stretches, and, as the symptoms of the condition begin to present very early on in the patient's life, many of my patients are young people, and so we tend to see lots of patients with cystic fibrosis finding these hospital visits frustrating. In fact, throughout the UK, about 80% of patients with cystic fibrosis who are hospitalised, report feeling at least minimal levels of depression.

M: How about young patients who aren't currently hospitalised? What can be challenging about their treatment?

F: Well, patients can be required to take around 30 pills a day to keep cystic fibrosis under control, so it's understandable that teenagers and young people, who just want to be free and independent, might resent this ordeal, if they think they can get away with it. One of the most difficult things we have to contend with is the fact that, if patients stop taking their medication, or doing their daily breathing treatments, their condition won't immediately worsen. Instead, it will gradually become more severe, until they contract a serious infection which puts their lives at risk.

M: So, what approaches do you use when treating patients with cystic fibrosis?

F: Well, we've found 'distraction therapy' to be extremely useful. We're incredibly lucky to have received a donation of a number of virtual reality headsets, following their success in a number of treatment trials. We use the virtual reality headsets to transport the patient to outdoor settings, often corresponding to the activities they're required to do with us. When they complete breathing exercises on a stationary bike, for example, the VR headsets display a virtual outdoor bike ride. Our patients find it helpful to pretend to be somewhere else during treatment, and it's often easier for us to administer breathing treatments to patients using these headsets, as they're more relaxed when they're not focused on the actuality of the test.

M: So what sorts of changes have you seen in your patients as a result of these methods?

F: One of my patients, a 24 year old man with cystic fibrosis who was in hospital waiting for a lung transplant… well, he found treatment very difficult at first. He was preoccupied by his need for a transplant, and frustrated by feelings of powerlessness. He would often resist treatment. We started using the virtual reality systems with him as soon as we got them, and, it took a while for him to get on board, but when he did, it was like someone had breathed new life into him. Not only did he stop hindering his treatment, he actually began to look forward to it. He's even started helping us to think about other ways we can improve the experiences of our patients, like improving social interaction.

M: Yes. I understand that there are difficulties involved in patient communication.

F: Mmmm… We're looking into the possibility of instant messaging functions between patients, and even virtual games that they can play against each other. Unfortunately, patients with cystic fibrosis have to be kept apart, to avoid cross-infection. It's just one more cross to bear for our patients, that they can't talk to those going through the same thing. Our patients get plenty of interaction with myself and the rest of the staff, but we'd like to make sure they have access to a network of fellow sufferers, too, for support and advice.

M: I see. That all sounds quite futuristic! Are there any other advances on the horizon, for the treatment of cystic fibrosis?

F: Well, there's a new drug that's been in the news recently, it's a combination of lumacaftor and ivacaftor, you might know it by the brand name Orkambi. The drug works by improving the level of water and salt in the body, thereby reducing the thick mucus that causes illness and respiratory issues in those with cystic fibrosis. Even more exciting and futuristic, though, is the possibility of gene therapy – where the genetic mutation that causes cystic fibrosis in individuals is replaced with a healthy gene. This would effectively cure those with the condition, and significantly extend the lives of thousands of people, and remove the need for lengthy stays in hospital.

Track 20

Hi everyone! My name's Dr Hubert Johnson, and I've been asked to speak to you about my experiences in the healthcare industry concerning something that effects all health professionals-improving efficiency.

It seems to be a given these days that practices will struggle with a lack of efficiency. We've actually found that this expectation, in and of itself, can reduce efficiency and increase delays even further! In a recent survey, when patients were asked why they arrived late to their appointments, 30% said that they had assumed that the previous appointment would run long. Patients expect to be kept waiting, and, to some extent, we expect that patients will be kept waiting, and so the first thing we need to address is our attitudes, and the attitudes of our patients.

So, let me start by telling you about the efficiency I observed in a practice I visited a couple of weeks ago. At this practise, patients could not make appointments online, but they could either phone up, or make an appointment in person. There were never more than 2 receptionists working in the morning, and the practice generally scheduled 80 appointments each day. Patients who were not attending a follow-up appointment were required to make their appointment on the day of. Can you imagine what that practice was like in the first couple of hours they were open? The receptionists were inundated by calls and walk-ins trying to schedule appointments.

As you can imagine, patients who had seen what the practice was like in the morning expected that if they didn't have the first slot of the day, they'd be delayed by at least 10 minutes. So, naturally, they arrived to their appointment 10 minutes late. One of the most important things you really must address in your practice, in order to improve efficiency, is the way you present your practice to patients. If they believe that you are always running late, guess what? They'll be running late too.

Now, let's think for a moment about what needs to be done on the patient's end before an appointment can take place. You might be thinking that there are only two steps to the process: one, the patient books an appointment, and two, the patient arrives at the practice in time for their appointment. Well, we healthcare professionals often forget that there's actually a step that comes before this: firstly, the patient must decide that their issue is significant enough to warrant an appointment.

So, about a decade ago, my practice was really struggling from a lack of efficiency. I was working extremely long hours to try to accommodate everyone, and I was becoming increasingly frustrated with conducting appointments that didn't seem strictly necessary. I got to thinking about how I might be able to help patients to reconsider their initial assumption when booking appointments, and to treat minor issues at home. At the same time, I did not want my patients to feel unsupported. I decided that I would begin to give weekly presentations in the evenings about self-care. As I tended to see a multitude of patients coming in for similar issues that they could actually treat themselves, each week I focused on a different common theme. The presentations lasted for just 1 hour, but I found that they resulted in 7 fewer unnecessary appointments each week.

These days, of course, I no longer have to give a physical presentation. Thanks to modern technology, I simply upload instructional videos to our practice's website. We also email these videos out to patients periodically. We can and should make use of technology as a tool in our practices, to help us to improve efficiency. However, it's important to note that while many, perhaps even the majority, of your patients will be capable of using technology to arrange their appointments, there are many people uncomfortable, or unable to use technology, so you must always make sure that these patients are accommodated, too. Providing your patients with more options, rather than replacing old options, is often the best practice for improving efficiency.

Now, let's move on to look at a practice that used technology in a surprising way...

PART THREE

The Reading Section

Reading Introduction

Section Overview

The OET Reading Test consists of three separate parts with a total of 42 questions, and takes 1 hour to complete.

The three different parts of the Reading Test are described below.

Part A of the Reading Test contains 4 texts on the same topic that a healthcare professional might use in the course of their work. You will have 15 minutes to answer 20 questions which cover a variety of question types about the information in the four texts.

Part B of the Reading Test contains 6 extracts from workplace communications in a healthcare setting. You should aim to spend roughly 10 minutes on this section.

Part C of the Reading Test contains 2 long passages providing information on different healthcare topics with 8 questions each. You should aim to spend roughly 35 minutes on this section.

Reading Strategies

- Unlike the OET Listening Test – where you must keep pace with the recording to avoid falling behind – you must pace yourself in the Reading Test. You should time yourself while you attempt the questions within this chapter.

- Make sure you are familiar with the Reading Test instructions in advance, so that on Test Day, you can focus on answering the questions.

- Familiarise yourself with the different parts of the Reading test, and be prepared for each question type. Use this chapter to build your knowledge of the different tasks in the Reading test, then assess your skills with the practice set of questions at the end of each part. Revisit and revise any questions you struggled with, identify what caused you to struggle with the question, and practise answering similar questions.

- Look out for the important words in the question that can help you to locate the information in the text.

CHAPTER 6

Reading Part A

LEARNING OBJECTIVES

By the end of this chapter, you will be able to:

- Scan the 4 texts to locate the information needed.
- Read sections of the 4 texts to find detailed meaning
- Practise strategies for answering Matching, Sentence Completion, and Short Answer questions.

Introduction

In Part A of the OET Reading Test, you have to answer 20 questions on 4 separate texts. You have 15 minutes to do this on Test Day. The texts in this section will be labelled **Text A** to **Text D**, and present information in different ways, but all relate to one health condition or type of treatment.

Strategies

Know the Instructions

You should make sure you are familiar with what you have to do before you take the test. The instructions for Reading Part A look like this:

TIME: 15 minutes

- Look at the four texts, **A – D**, in the **Text Booklet**.
- For each question, **1 – 20**, look through the texts, **A – D**, to find the relevant information.
- Write your answers on the spaces provided in this **Question Paper**.
- Answer all the questions within the 15-minute time limit.

Know the Format

In Part A of the Reading Test, you need to look at the 4 texts provided across two pages of your test booklet. The 4 texts in this section are examples of a variety of text types you might find in the workplace – including at least one that presents visual or tabular information, such as: a flow chart, table, or diagram. Other texts in Part A include information in paragraphs and bullet-pointed lists. Some of the texts in this section contain numbers, but you are not required to make any calculations.

The 4 texts in Reading Part A test your ability to consult and understand practical reference documents for specific conditions and treatments, for example, one of the texts might outline the correct procedure to follow when a patient has a broken arm. Don't worry if at first the topic of the texts are unfamiliar to you, you will not need to have prior knowledge of the specific condition or treatment discussed in the texts for Reading Part A. Simply focus on finding the word or phrase in the relevant text that allows you to answer each individual question.

When you begin Part A, you should start by looking briefly at each of the four texts in the test booklet to understand the type of information being provided in each text. You should spend only a short time looking at the 4 texts before answering the questions, as the first task will help you to understand the information provided in the 4 texts.

Exercise

Briefly look at the four texts on the following 2 pages, then answer questions 1 – 5 as quickly as you can.

Hypertension: Texts

Text A

> The medications used to treat high blood pressure fall under one of the following categories describing their mechanism of action:
>
> - ACE-inhibitor
> - Angiotensin-II antagonist
> - Calcium-channel blocker
> - Thiazide-type diuretic
>
> Which medication a patient receives depends on their age and ethnicity. Black patients of African or Caribbean descent are known to have higher risk of hypertension. Whenever a patient's treatment regime fails to work, it is stepped-up by adding an additional medication of a different category.

Text B

Controlling High Blood Pressure

- Advise patients to stop smoking; offer advice for help and counselling. Patients can use nicotine aids and join local 'stop smoking' schemes. If unable to quit smoking, encourage them to reduce daily cigarette consumption.
- Patients must not drink alcohol to excess and stick to weekly alcohol limits, which are 14 Units per week MAXIMUM for both males and females.
- Encourage regular exercise, at least 150 minutes of moderate aerobic activity (such as walking, cycling, swimming) per week, including strength exercises on at least two days per week.
- Recommend a balanced and healthy diet, low in saturated fats and sugars. Patients should opt for lean proteins, brown carbs, and fruit and vegetables.
- Advise those with high blood pressure to purchase a blood pressure monitor to use at home so that they can measure blood pressure regularly.
- Patients should keep a blood pressure log and take to each check-up appointment.
- Provide strategies to help minimise stress and anxiety at home and at work. Offer advice about help and counselling, recommend local services for stress, anxiety, or depression.

Text C

The following are indicators of high blood pressure:

- Severe, sudden and recurring headaches
- Frequent nose-bleeds
- Visual changes, such as blurred vision
- Dizziness
- Shortness of breath
- Chest pain
- Numbness

High blood pressure is one of the biggest risk factors for heart disease and stroke. It is a worldwide issue and is becoming increasingly common. There would be a significant reduction in the incidence of heart disease and stroke in the UK if all patients with high blood pressure made lifestyle changes and took steps to lower and control it.

Text D

The table below shows the systolic and diastolic values for normal and abnormal blood pressure.

Category:	Systolic Pressure (mmHg):		Diastolic Pressure (mmHg):
Hypotension	70–89	or	40–59
Normal Blood Pressure	90–119	and	60–79
Prehypertension	120–139	or	80–89
Stage 1 (Mild) Hypertension	140–159	or	90–99
Stage 2 (Moderate) Hypertension	160–179	or	100–109
Stage 3 (Severe) Hypertension	180–209	or	110–119

1.   For each of the four texts, **A – D**, briefly summarise the information given.

2.   Look in **Text A** to find who has an increased risk of high blood pressure.

3.   Look in **Text D** to find which category of blood pressure a diastolic measure of 85 mmHG would belong to?

4.   Look in **Text B** to find what type of exercise patients should do two times each week?

5.   Look in **Text C** to find what would happen if patients with high blood pressure made an effort to lower it.

In Part A of the Reading Test, you need to answer questions using information in the texts as you have just done in this exercise. However, unlike the previous exercise, on Test Day you will not be told which text to find the information in, so you need to be prepared to scan all four texts to find the relevant information, before you can complete the question.

The questions in this part of the test don't follow the order of the texts. Each task in this part of the test operates in a different way, and each task will refer to all 4 texts.

Before you scan the texts for answers, however, you should pay attention to the words in the question, as these could suggest which text you will find the correct answer in. For each question, underline the most important words or phrases to help you scan the texts to find the answers.

Identify the Question Types

In Part A of the Reading Test there are 4 possible task types: Matching, Short Answer, Sentence Completion and Note Completion. The first task will always be Matching, and this task will always be followed by 2 of the other 3 task types. In Part A, the 20 questions will be split across 3 or 4 groups of questions.

Questions 6–25 on the following pages can be answered by referring to the 4 texts about the thyroid on pages 71 to 74.

Matching Questions

The first task in Reading Part A always asks you to identify which text contains the information. You should always answer these questions first, as they will help you to gain an understanding of the content within each text.

To answer these questions, look at the information given in the question. The questions will avoid repeating words and phrases exactly as they appear in the texts, so you will need to understand the meaning of the question, and find the matching information in one of the passages. The questions in this section ask you to identify which text contains a particular type of information or information about a particular aspect of the condition or issue. For example, a Matching Question might ask 'Which text provides information about identifying delirium in patients?' To answer these questions, you need to understand the general meaning of the 4 texts, rather than the specific details.

Exercise

Answer questions **6 – 11** using the 4 texts on pages 71 to 74. You should complete these questions in 3 minutes.

In which text can you find information about...

6. identifying the risk of malignant cancer of the thyroid?

7. which patients are suitable for a thyroidectomy?

8. the symptoms of patients receiving insufficient treatment?

9. changing the dosage of thyroid medication?

10. assessing the thyroid function in those taking L-thyroxine?

11. possible complications involved in thyroid removal procedure?

Short Answer Questions

To answer Short Answer questions, you need to locate the correct word or short phrase from the texts. You will have to write the answer to these questions using only the information given in the texts. Short Answer questions will require you to look at the four texts in more detail than you did for Matching questions, as the answers to Short Answer questions might be found in a single sentence in one of the texts. These questions will often include specific words, such as types of medication, treatment or reactions in patients, that you can look for in the four texts to find where this type of information in presented. Once you've found the information, you need to understand the type of word or phrase you need to answer the question. Look at the question to understand what type of information is being asked for; for example, a question that asks 'What should patients suffering from fever be given?' could be answered with a type of medication, a beverage, or an item. The question could not, on the other hand, be answered with a number alone, or a type of illness. When you're struggling to find the answer to the question, it can be helpful to narrow down the type of answer you need, and look for the possible answers in the relevant text.

Make sure you copy the words exactly, and do not include words or phrases that are not present in the text. The answer will generally require 1 to 3 words from the text. Keep your answers short, and avoid including unnecessary information, as it may lead the assessor to believe that you do not understand the text fully, or are not sure of the correct answer.

IMPROVE YOUR SCORE

If you're confident you've identified the information in one of the texts, without checking the other texts, write your answer down and move on.

Exercise

Answer questions **12 – 16** using the 4 texts on pages 71 to 74. For each answer, use a word or short phrase from the text. Each answer may include words, numbers or both. You should complete these questions in 5 minutes.

12. What will the level of FT4 be in patients undergoing thyroxine replacement therapy?

_____

13. What should patients who are taking L-thyroxine do if they notice arrhythmia and mood swings?

_____

14. Which type of thyroidectomy has an increased chance of morbidity?

_____

15. Test results for a patient with subclinical hyperthyroidism will show what level of FT3?

_____

16. What can be tested for using a commercially available kit?

_____

Sentence Completion

To answer Sentence Completion questions, you need to fill the gaps in each sentence with a word or short phrase from one of the texts.

The process for answering these questions is similar to that used for Short Answer questions. Look at the words in the sentence that are likely to guide you to the information in the text, scan the text for these words until you find the information, and identify the word or short phrase that is most likely to complete the sentence.

Before completing the sentence, read the sentence to yourself (in your head, not out loud) with your answer, to confirm that the sentence makes sense using the words you have chosen. If it does, complete the sentence. If it does not make sense, read the relevant piece of information more closely, and choose another word or short phrase.

IMPROVE YOUR SCORE

The questions in this section are not given in the order that the four texts appear, so if you've just answered a question with information from the third text, this does not mean that the next question will be in the final text. Make sure to check all four of the texts to find the answer.

Exercise

Answer questions **17 – 21** using a word or short phrase from the 4 texts on pages 71 to 74. Each answer may include words, numbers or both. You should complete these questions in 5 minutes.

17. If thyroid function tests indicate that TSH has **(17)** _____, this could suggest heterophile antibodies.

18. Following a thyroidectomy, if the patient experiences aphonia, this suggests injury to the **(18)** _____.

19. If tests reveal that the BRAF V600E mutation is present, it is extremely likely that the patient has **(19)** _____.

20. During a thyroidectomy, the endoscope is inserted into a cut made in the **(20)** _____.

21. To optimise hypothyroidism treatment, **(21)** _____ can be used to detect euthyroidism, once the current treatment is stopped.

Thyroid: Texts

Text A

Diagnosis of Hypothyroidism in Patients Taking L-thyroxine

Patients frequently take thyroid hormone with an inadequate diagnosis of hypothyroidism, this is clinically relevant and should be addressed to optimise treatment. Presenting complaints include fatigue, weight gain, and oligo menorrhea. If the patient and doctor establish that the diagnosis was not complete – the best approach is to stop treatment for 5 weeks. L-thyroxine and desiccated thyroid extract are the most common treatment options. After stopping treatment, serum T_4 and TSH concentrations will indicate euthyroidism or a primary hypothyroid state.

Carry out tests 10-14 days after stopping drug therapy and analyse the results for physiological hypothyroidism from suppression of the pituitary-thyroid axis by the exogenous hormone.

Alternative approach: halve the L-thyroxine dose and assess thyroid function after 5 weeks.

Patients taking an excessive amount of L-thyroxine may experience the following symptoms:

- mood changes/swings
- tremor
- bone pain

- arrhythmia
- chest pain
- diarrhoea

Advise patients to be aware of these symptoms, and to seek immediate medical help if more than one of these symptoms occurs.

Text B

MINIMALLY INVASIVE VIDEO-ASSISTED THYROIDECTOMY

Procedure:

- Usually undertaken with the patient under general anaesthesia.
- Small incision made above the sternal notch
- Endoscope inserted through incision
- Dissection of thyroid lobe undertaken
- Operative space maintained using external retraction
    o Do not use gas insufflation
- Care must be taken to identify and preserve recurrent laryngeal nerve

Safety:

- Postoperative morbidity rates, meta-analysis of 9 studies:
    o 10% (29 out of 289) for minimally invasive video-assisted thyroidectomy
    o 14% (42 out of 292) for conventional, open thyroidectomy
- Superficial laryngeal nerve injury reported in 2% (5 out of 300) of patients
    o Can lead to:
        • Weakened voice (hoarseness)
        • Loss of voice (aphonia)
        • Problems with the respiratory tract

Training:

- Minimally invasive video-assisted thyroidectomy requires skills additional to those of conventional, open thyroid surgery.
- Adequate training is important for surgeons using the minimally invasive procedure
- The procedure is only suitable for a minority of patients with thyroid disease
    o Those requiring surgery
    o Those with thyroid glands of an appropriate size

Text C

BRAF V600E Mutation Testing for Thyroid Cancer

Mutation testing should be undertaken to avoid unnecessary surgery and reduce the number of surgical procedures for patients with suspected thyroid cancer.

- Fine needle aspiration is the most common method to obtain thyroid tissue samples
- Cytological examination cannot distinguish between benign and malignant neoplasms
    - o If the biopsy is positive – the affected lobe is surgically removed
    - o The sample undergoes a pathological microscopic examination
    - o If the testing indicates cancer – the remainder of the thyroid gland is removed
- A test for a BRAF V600E mutation can be performed using a commercially available testing kit
- The BRAF V600E mutation has more than 99% specificity for thyroid cancer
    - o A positive result means that there is more than 99% chance the cancer is malignant
- This makes it possible to remove the thyroid in one operation rather than two

Text D

Thyroid Function Test Results and Analysis

TSH	FT$_4$	FT$_3$	Clinical
Decreased	Normal	Normal	– thyroxine treatment/ingestion – subclinical hyperthyroidism – drugs: steroid, dopamine – non-thyroidal illness
Decreased or Normal	Decreased or Normal	Decreased or Normal	– non-thyroidal illness – early phase post-treatment for hyperthyroidism – pituitary disease – congenital TSH deficiency
Increased	Normal	Normal	– subclinical hypothyroidism – heterophile antibody (interferes with TSH assay) – erratic compliance with thyroxine therapy – malabsorption of thyroxine in previously stable patient – drugs: amiodarone, cholestyramine, iron – recovery phase of non-thyroidal illness – TSH resistance
Normal or Increased	Normal or Increased	Normal or Increased	– drugs: heparin, amiodarone – anti-iodothyronine antibodies, anti-TSH antibodies – familial dysalbuminaemic hypothyroxinaemia (FDH) – thyroxine replacement therapy (including non-compliance) – non-thyroidal illness, acute psychological disorders – TSH-secreting pituitary tumour – resistance to thyroid hormone

Remember, you only have 15 minutes to answer all 20 questions in Part A, so you must use your time wisely. By the time you get to the different sets of questions, such as Short Answer, Note Completion and Incomplete Sentences, you should be familiar enough with the texts that you can identify the text that the information is likely to appear in, just by reading the question. When this is the case, check the text to confirm, find the answer, and move on to the next question. Working briskly and efficiently are the keys to succeeding on Test Day.

Reading Part A Practice Set

TIME: 15 minutes

- Look at the four texts, **A – D**, on pages 78 – 81.
- For each question, **1 – 20**, look through the texts, **A – D**, to find the relevant information.
- Write your answers in the spaces provided in this **Question Paper**.
- Answer all the questions within the 15-minute time limit.

Anaemia: Questions

Questions 1 – 6

For each question below, decide which text (A, B, C or D) the information comes from.

You may use any letter more than once.

In which text can you find information about . . .

1. treating patients with anaemia?

2. the symptoms of hypoxia?

3. methods used to identify anaemic patients?

4. the different types of anaemia?

5. the levels of haemoglobin in a woman with anaemia?

6. how red blood cell size affects anaemia?

Questions 7 – 14

Answer the questions below. For each answer, use a word or short phrase from the text. Each answer may include words, numbers or both.

7. What should vegan patients with vitamin deficiency anaemia be encouraged to add to their diets?

    _____

8. If there is a decreased number of young red blood cells, what type of anaemia is being dealt with?

    _____

9. How will a patient's breathing sound when experiencing a significant reduction of oxygen in the body's tissues?

    _____

10. A male with anaemia must have less than what percentage of red blood cells?

    _____

11. What is an increase in the number of reticulocytes an indication of?

    _____

12. What reduces the amount of red blood cells in some patients?

    _____

13. What should be treated in anaemic patients, after identifying the cause?

    _____

14. How are the different types of anaemia most commonly distinguished?

    _____

Questions 15 – 20

Complete the sentences below by using a word or short phrase from the text. Each answer may include words, numbers or both.

15. Anaemia caused by **(15)**_____ should be treated with a blood transfusion.

16. Patients suffering from hypoxia and chest pain are likely to also have a **(16)**_____.

17. If **(17)**_____ is functioning properly, high reticulocyte anaemia is likely to be present.

18. A number of tests may be necessary to diagnose anaemia, due to the difficulties involved in measuring **(18)**_____.

19. Patients with anaemia caused by **(19)**_____ should be instructed to adjust their diet.

20. When identifying the type of aetiology, **(20)**_____ of the patient should be considered, in addition to laboratory studies.

Anaemia: Texts

Text A

Anaemia is defined as an overall decrease in red blood cell mass. There are many varying causes of anaemia, which all present with some general symptoms. Anaemia results in a lack of red blood cells in the blood. Because it is the haemoglobin in red blood cells that carries oxygen from the lungs to the rest of the body, a decrease in red blood cells results in less oxygen going into the tissues. This causes a state known as hypoxia, or reduced oxygen in body tissues.

The common symptoms of all anaemias are those of hypoxia:

- Weakness, fatigue, difficult or laboured breathing
- Pale skin
- Headache and light-headedness
- Chest pain (if the patient already has a disease of the arteries supplying the heart)

Text B

There are many classification systems to differentiate anaemias. The most commonly used is based on the size of the red blood cell. Anaemias with red blood cells that are smaller than normal are known as microcytic anaemias. If the anaemia has normally sized red blood cells, it is referred to as a normocytic anaemia. Finally, if the red blood cells are too big, it is known as a macrocytic anaemia. Normocytic anaemias are further broken up into whether or not there is an increased number of young red blood cells (a.k.a. reticulocytes), which is an indication if the bone marrow is working properly—for example, if the red blood cells are being destroyed (haemolysis), there should be higher reticulocytes because there is no effect on the bone marrow's ability to produce new cells.

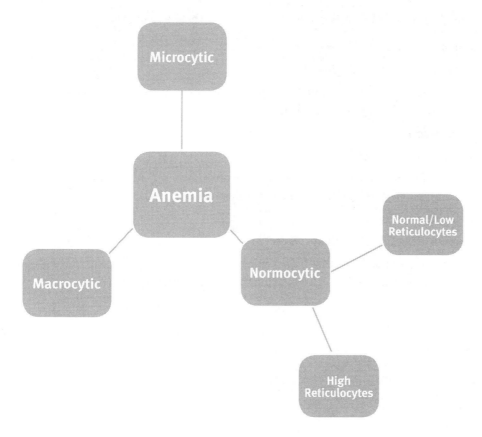

Text C

While there are many different causes of anaemia, laboratory studies and unique features of the patient can be used to help differentiate between various aetiologies.

Laboratory studies used to diagnose anaemia include:

- Haemoglobin (Hb)—a measure of the protein that transports oxygen in the red blood cell
- Haematocrit (Hct)—a measure of the percentage of red blood cells in the blood
- Red blood cell amount (erythrocyte count)—a measure of the number of red blood cells in the blood

A general diagnosis of anaemia can be determined by the following values:

- Haemoglobin level
  - o Males: less than 13.5 g/dL
  - o Females: less than 12.5 g/dL (women have a generally lower haemoglobin because of blood loss during the monthly menstrual cycle)
- Haematocrit
  - o Males: less than 45% red blood cells
  - o Females: less than 37% red blood cells (women have a generally lower haematocrit because of blood loss during the monthly menstrual cycle)
- Red blood cell amount
  - o Male: less than 4.7 million cells/mL
  - o Female: less than 4.2 million cells/mL (women have a generally lower red blood cell amount because of blood loss during the monthly menstrual cycle)

While these laboratory tests are good estimates of the red blood cell mass, they are not perfect. Red blood cell mass is very difficult to measure, and therefore these laboratory tests are used together to assess whether or not someone has anaemia.

Text D

The treatment of anaemia depends heavily on the type of anaemia that the patient is experiencing. However, there are several overarching goals of treatment.

1. If possible, treat the underlying cause of the red blood cell loss.

   a. For example, if the patient has anaemia because of blood loss, give a blood transfusion.

2. Identify and treat any complications that have occurred because of the anaemia.

3. Educate the patient on how to manage their anaemia.

   a. For example, a patient with anaemia because of iron deficiency can supplement their treatment with iron rich foods, such as leafy green vegetables.

   b. Alternatively, a patient with anaemia caused by vitamin deficiency should be advised to increase their intake of folic acid and B-12. Note that patients who follow vegetarian or vegan diets may struggle to meet B-12 requirements, so eating fortified foods and using supplements should be advised.

Answers

1	**A** – Medication options for patients with high blood pressure. **B** – Advice to give patients with high blood pressure to control their condition **C** – symptoms of high blood pressure **D** – systolic and diastolic levels for normal and abnormal blood pressure
2	Black patients of African or Caribbean descent
3	Prehypertension
4	strength exercises
5	There would be a significant reduction in the incidence of heart disease and stroke
6	C
7	B
8	A
9	D
10	B
11	B
12	normal or increased
13	seek immediate medical help
14	(conventional) open thyroidectomy
15	normal
16	a BRAF V600E mutation
17	increased
18	superficial laryngeal nerve
19	malignant cancer
20	sternal notch
21	serum T4 and TSH concentrations

Practice Set

1	D
2	A
3	C
4	B
5	C
6	B
7	fortified foods (and supplements)
8	low reticulocytes
9	laboured
10	45
11	reticulocytes
12	menstrual cycle
13	complications
14	size of the red blood cell
15	blood loss
16	disease of the arteries
17	bone marrow
18	iron deficiency
19	chest pain
20	unique features

CHAPTER 7

Reading Part B

LEARNING OBJECTIVES

By the end of this chapter, you will be able to:

- Understand the different reading text types.
- Read the text carefully to identify the correct answer.
- Practise strategies for answering Reading Part B questions.

Introduction

Part B of the Reading Test in OET is very similar to Part B of the Listening Test. In Reading Part B, you will read 6 different extracts from documents giving background information for healthcare professionals, and answer one question about each extract. You have 45 minutes to complete Parts B and C of the Reading Test. You should allow roughly 10 minutes to complete this section so you leave yourself enough time to complete Part C. This means you should aim to spend on average 1 minute 30 seconds to complete each Part B question, although you may find some questions quicker to answer while others may take more time.

Strategies

Know the Instructions

You should make sure you are familiar with what you will be asked to do on Test Day. The instructions for Part B of the Reading Test will look like this:

In this part of the test, there are six short extracts relating to the work of health professionals. For **questions 1 to 6**, choose the answer (**A**, **B** or **C**) which you think fits best according to the text.

Write your answers on the separate **Answer Sheet**.

Know the Settings

Reading Part B contains 6 different healthcare texts. The texts in this part of the test are generic hospital-based texts which can be used and understood by any of the 12 healthcare professions covered by the test.

The texts that you will see in this section of the test represent the types of texts and documents that healthcare professionals will often refer to for specific reasons. Rather than focusing on technical medical information that you might find in a textbook, for instance, these documents will cover guidelines, policies and procedures. They might remind healthcare professionals of the best practice to follow in a given circumstance, or updates to a data storage system, or even instruct employees how to use machinery. Part B texts will generally be made up of extracts from the following test types:

- **Notices**
- **Emails**
- **Manuals**
- **Memos**
- **Guidelines**

To answer as many questions in this section correctly as possible, you need to focus your efforts on understanding the main point of the information provided in each of the texts.

Scan the Question

Unlike the Listening Test, the OET Reading Test does not provide additional time to look through the questions before answering them, so you should factor this into your total time. You should aim to answer 6 questions in roughly 10 minutes, so don't spend too long on any one question. If you can't find the answer, move on to the next question and come back to this one at the end.

In this section of the test, there are three different question types. We'll go through each question type now, and provide examples for each question type.

Main Idea

These questions ask for the main idea of the piece of information. To answer these questions, you will need to assess what the main point is of what is being communicated.

Exercise

Take 4 minutes and 30 seconds to answer questions **1 – 3** below.

1. The policy document tells us that a healthcare professional's

    (**A**) duty to care for a patient continues after a referral.

    (**B**) ability to look after a patient should be decided by superiors.

    (**C**) obligation to check up on transfers does not apply to all patients.

CONTINUITY AND COORDINATION OF CARE

All healthcare professionals must be involved in the safe transfer of patients between each other and social care providers. This includes:

*   Sharing all relevant information with colleagues that are involved with your patient's care, both inside and outside the team, including when the care handover is done at the end of duty, and when care is delegated or referred to other health or social care providers.

*   When possible, check that a named team or clinician has appropriately taken over responsibility when your role has ended in providing a patient's care. This is most important in vulnerable patients who do not have capacity.

When care is transferred or delegated to another healthcare professional, it is your responsibility to ensure that the person providing care has the appropriate skills, qualifications and experience to provide adequately safe care for the patient.

---

2. The guidelines inform us that physical restraints

    (**A**) can only be administered to patients by qualified staff.

    (**B**) must be applied before patients become aggressive.

    (**C**) should only be used on patients as a last resort.

ASSESSING PHYSICAL RESTRAINTS

We first advise providers to verbally de-escalate and offer medications as a method of calming an agitated patient down. However, if these do not work and the patient becomes violent, a standard protocol for physical restraints should be followed. Trained personnel should carry out the actual action of physically restraining the patient and a bed with restraints should be prepared ahead of time. Medications should be drawn up in IM form and be ready to be given once the patient has been physically restrained. A physician should then assess the patient, first debriefing staff on the situation that caused the patient to be placed in restraints and then speak to the patient personally to determine their understanding of the same events. Cardiopulmonary status and restraint tightness must be assessed and the patient's level of pain and distress documented.

---

3. The guidelines advise physicians on

(A) seeking advice from others.

(B) receiving authorisation for care.

(C) referring patients to different departments.

CALLING A CONSULT

No physician can handle every patient by themselves. No matter the specialty, there will come a time where you need to reach out for additional help. If you're working at an outpatient office, you'll look to a specialist in a different institution. If you're working inside the hospital, you'll call a particular service with a consult. Different institutions have different protocols on how to call the consult, but at the very core, you will need to present the patient to the physician you've consulted. You should start by introducing yourself and your role on the treatment team. Give a short summary of the patient, their medical history, why they're in the hospital and what's happened so far. You should then go into the reason you're consulting the specialist and what you're looking for – whether it's treatment recommendations, a procedure, or to arrange a service transfer. Conclude by asking if they have any other questions that you can help answer.

IMPROVE YOUR SCORE

The answer choices will avoid repeating words or phrases from the text. As such, it is important to think about the overall meaning of the extract, and choose the answer choice that best corresponds to this. The extracts in Reading Part B are short, so give yourself time to read through the entire text, using the question to direct your understanding, before you consider the answer choices.

Detail

Detail questions will ask you to answer a question about a specific part of the text. They will often include words in the question that you can use to skim the text for the relevant information.

Exercise

Take 6 minutes to answer questions **4 – 7** below.

4. What point does the training manual make about confidential documents?

    Ⓐ They must not be consulted in an open area.

    Ⓑ They must only be shared via work email.

    Ⓒ They must be destroyed after use.

ENSURING PATIENT PRIVACY

Patient privacy is legally governed by HIPAA, which establishes strict standards for healthcare providers when sharing patient information. Every hospital will have guidelines healthcare employees must follow to avoid committing an HIPAA violation, which can result in termination from employment and/or severe fines. Employees must avoid talking about identifiable patient information with other people that are not involved in their care. This also includes discussing patient details in a public setting like a hallway or elevator. When sending information about patients to other providers, it is important to use secure forms of transmission such as hospital email and fax. Avoid easy but unprotected methods like texting or personal email. Dispose of any identifiable information in specially marked bins for later incineration.

---

5. What should staff with open cuts exposed to a bloodborne viral illness do?

    (A) avoid contact with other staff.

    (B) prevent a scab from forming.

    (C) disinfect and cover the wound.

EXTRACT FROM GUIDELINES: POST-EXPOSURE PROPHYLAXIS FOR HIV

When working with patients with suspected or confirmed HIV infection or other bloodborne viral illnesses, medical staff must remember that they are at risk of inoculation injury, and take necessary precautions to prevent infection.

It is important that strict guidelines are adhered to and rapid action taken post-exposure, in order to reduce potential risk of infection post-incident, control spread, and prevent future incidents. Exposures are defined as percutaneous inoculation via a needlestick injury, or a splash of potentially infected body fluids/blood into mucous membranes (such as eyes or mouth) or an open wound. Immediate action should be taken to wash the injury or exposed region with copious amounts of water; any wounds should be encouraged to bleed, and prevented from beginning to clot before the area has been cleaned. Senior members of staff should be informed immediately, and the Occupational Health department contacted. All cases will be dealt with confidentially and all blood samples taken from the affected member of staff will be labelled anonymously. An Incident Form should be completed urgently. Occupational Health will rapidly arrange contact with, and testing of, the source patient.

---

6. The guidelines inform us that codeine can cause side effects in patients

(A) who suffer from opioid addiction.

(B) who take it together with morphine.

(C) who have a particular genetic makeup.

CODEINE AND ULTRA-RAPID METABOLISERS

Codeine is a widely used opioid analgesic used to treat mild to moderate pain. The ability to metabolise codeine to morphine can vary considerably between individuals. Codeine has a very low affinity for opioid receptors and its analgesic effect is due to its conversion to morphine. The hepatic CYP2D6 enzyme that metabolises a quarter of all prescribed drugs, including codeine, regulates this process.

Individuals who have two or more functional copies of the CYP2D6 gene are ultra-rapid metabolisers - able to metabolise codeine to morphine more rapidly and completely. Even at normal doses, individuals who are ultra-rapid metabolisers may have life-threatening or fatal respiratory depression, or experience signs of overdose. Individuals with no active copies of CYP2D6 ("poor metabolisers") show reduced morphine levels. In this scenario, alternative pain management strategies must be established.

Healthcare professionals and prescribers are encouraged to educate patients about possible side effects associated with codeine use.

---

7. The guidelines inform us that incisional hernias

(A) are caused by surgery.

(B) form when patients cut themselves.

(C) occur more frequently than other hernias.

GUIDELINES: INCISIONAL HERNIA

In 12–15% of abdominal operations, incisional hernias occur post-operatively. An incisional hernia passes through an incision previously made during surgery, when the closure of abdominal tissues fails to heal properly. Be sure to cover during check-ups: incisional hernias are the second most common type of hernia.

Check for hernia

-   Look for abnormal protrusion of tissue or organ through the cavity in which it is situated.
-   Remember that hernias are most common in the abdomen, but can also appear in the upper thighs and groin region.

Remember that the major risk with incisional hernias is strangulation: the organ in the hernia devascularises and the tissue degenerates. This must be identified at the earliest opportunity – delay can lead to septicaemia and shock.

Treatment is mostly surgical: a mesh can be used to strengthen the area. Otherwise, open and keyhole repairs remain an option, however, better outcomes have been reported with the use of mesh repairs.

IMPROVE YOUR SCORE

The question can help you to identify the type of text. Generally, Part B multiple-choice questions will help to understand the text by explaining the type of text, or where you might find it. Use this information to help you to understand the text, for example, if the text is an extract of a policy update for healthcare staff, it's likely to discuss recent changes to practices and protocol.

Purpose

Purpose questions require you to choose the answer that best explains the point of the text. Think about why the text was written, what should healthcare professionals reading the text do as a result of reading it?

Exercise

Take 4 minutes and 30 seconds to answer questions **8 – 10** below.

8. The main purpose of the guidelines is to advise staff on

   (A) the procedure to follow when fitting an IV.

   (B) how to check for issues with IV infusions.

   (C) what to do before administering an IV.

PROCEDURAL GUIDELINES FOR SET-UP AND ADMINISTRATION OF INTRAVENOUS FLUIDS

Intravenous (IV) fluids are infused directly into the veins of patients via a cannula in cases of severe dehydration, electrolyte imbalance, blood loss, and in surgery. Intravenous lines can also be used for administration of drugs directly into the blood of a patient, resulting in faster action. The guidelines below illustrate the correct procedure for setting up and administering IV therapy.

Firstly, always check that the fluid bag is not damaged and that the liquid inside it is clear. Secondly, there have been reports of incomplete patient notes, so it is crucial that you check for details such as fluid type and expiration date and record these in the patient notes immediately. Thirdly, it is vital that all clinical staff introduce themselves with their full name and role to all patients they engage with; only after confirming patient details and obtaining their consent should one begin the IV set-up. Finally, be extra diligent when calculating the drip rate as to avoid any errors. Feel comfortable to approach a fellow colleague for assistance if uncertain at any stage.

---

9.   The purpose of the email is to advise paediatricians to be

(A) mindful that parents may not always agree with the proposed treatment.

(B) aware that even minor illnesses can be distressing for parents.

(C) understanding and patient when explaining conditions to children.

For the attention of all paediatricians:

As a paediatrician, one must always remember that the patients are not the doctor's only concern; we must also factor in the anxious parents worried about their child. This can be an additional challenge for staff in a department that is already busy and stressful, but a duty which must not be neglected. Parents who seek paediatric care for minor conditions are not intentionally impinging on medical care for those patients who more urgently need it. Therefore, time should be spent speaking to these parents and offering reassurance and support as appropriate, rather than ignoring them or making them a last priority. Ten to fifteen minutes spent in conversation with these families will save much more time in the long-run and prevent countless bleeps and calls from them, which could otherwise have been avoided. In addition, it is vital to be aware of alternative potential causes for the parental anxiety that could be rooted in past events and experiences, or caused by problems in their personal life.

10. What is the email from the admin team asking front-line staff to do over the next 6 months?

   (A) Charge a fee to patients who cancel their appointments three times.

   (B) Call patients with a reminder 24 hours prior to their appointment.

   (C) Inform patients of the changes to be implemented.

To all front-line medical staff,

Recently, we have been noticing a steady increase in no-show appointments at the practice. Previously, we did not have a concrete policy on cancellation deadlines or missed appointment fees. Given that no-show appointments not only take up valuable time from our providers, but also prevent another patient from utilising these time slots, it is in our best interest to discourage patients from missing their appointment. Going forward, office staff will call every patient at least 48 hours before their appointment to remind them of the date and time of their appointment. If the patient cancels within 24 hours of their appointment time, office staff will make a note in the patient's chart. If the patient has more than three such cancellations, he or she will then be issued with a $25 fee to reschedule the appointment. Patients who are using medical insurance are exempt from this fee and instead should have their chart forwarded to a provider for further evaluation. We understand that this new policy may result in some difficulties for staff, so we will allow fees to be waived in extreme circumstances. We will also set the start date of this policy six months from today's date, so all patients will have sufficient time to be informed of the new rules. Please make sure that all patients are aware of these changes at the end of each appointment.

Many thanks,

The admin team

Part B of the Reading Test is designed to assess your ability to scan and select relevant information from healthcare texts that you are likely to encounter while working in your profession. Practise for this section of the test by reading through instructive materials and making notes on what is being explained. Take note of the purpose of any emails or communications you receive in English, and pay attention to signs and notices in English, as these will often use similar language and settings to those used in this part of the test.

Reading Part B Practice Set

Part B

In this part of the test, there are six short extracts relating to the work of health professionals. For **questions 1 to 6**, choose the answer (**A**, **B** or **C**) which you think fits best according to the text.

Write your answers on the separate **Answer Sheet**.

1. Why is epinephrine added to Lidocaine injections?

   A to numb the area

   B to prolong the effects

   C to reduce patient discomfort

PREPARATION OF INJECTION

Lidocaine is a local anesthetic that is often injected subcutaneously before minor medical procedures such as laceration repair, excisional biopsy, and hormone implantation. A key step to prepare for this procedure is clearing a suitable workspace and obtaining any necessary supplies. First, be sure to check with your provider about the concentration and mixture of Lidocaine to be used. Epinephrine is often included to constrict local blood vessels for longer duration, but can increase the risk of causing ischemia in areas with poor blood supply (fingers, ears, toes). Sodium bicarbonate can also be added to avoid pain during injection due to Lidocaine's acidic pH. Be sure to obtain the proper sized needle and syringe, which will be dependent on the location of the injection and the size of the area requiring anesthesia, respectively.

---

2. The policy document on collateral information offers advice to staff about how to

    (A) gather information from colleagues about specific patients.

    (B) collect information about patients from their friends and relatives.

    (C) inform patients and their carers about recent diagnoses over the phone.

POLICY REMINDER: COLLECTING COLLATERAL INFORMATION

Collateral information is an important factor in determining appropriate disposition for psychiatric patients in the Emergency Department. Often, patients with psychiatric complaints are unable to accurately or thoroughly describe their medical history, baseline condition, or events leading up to their arrival at the hospital. Thus, it becomes imperative to contact those who might know the patient best or were in the patient's company prior to their arrival. Contact information can be obtained from the patient themselves, persons accompanying the patient, or the medical record. When initiating contact, confirm the other person's identity before revealing the patient's name or the reason you are speaking with them. If you reach voicemail and the answering machine does not clearly identify the person you are looking for, do not reveal any information about the patient – simply state your name, number, position, and whom you are requesting a callback from.

---

3.   When dealing with patients with symptoms of peripheral arterial disease, staff
     should

(A)   look for signs of swelling in the upper body.

(B)   confirm that the patient has a history of poor diet.

(C)   identify the cause through physical examination and tests.

ASSESSING AND MANAGING PERIPHERAL ARTERIAL DISEASE

Staff should assess patients who have symptoms suggestive of peripheral arterial
disease or diabetes with non-healing wounds for the presence of peripheral
arterial disease.

- Ask about the presence of intermittent claudication and critical limb
  ischaemia

- Examine the lower limbs for evidence of critical limb ischaemia

- Examine pulses in the lower limbs: femoral, popliteal and feet

- Measure the ankle brachial pressure index

Imaging is possible for patients with peripheral arterial disease: duplex
ultrasound is the first-line imaging technique. If patients require additional
imaging, contrast-enhanced magnetic resonance angiography is used. If this is
contraindicated or not possible, use computed tomography angiography instead.

Lifestyle changes are the first-line treatment for peripheral arterial disease, this
includes: smoking cessation, better control of diabetes, better management of
hypertension, management of high cholesterol, in combination with antiplatelet
drugs. Finally, regular exercise has shown to beneficially revascularise tissues in
those with claudication.

---

4.   The guidelines on alcohol withdrawal treatment informs healthcare professionals about

   Ⓐ   determining the quantity of medication required.

   Ⓑ   reducing the dosage as the symptoms improve.

   Ⓒ   various types of drugs to prescribe to patients.

GUIDELINES: ALCOHOL WITHDRAWAL TREATMENT

Alcohol withdrawal can present as a life-threatening emergency and requires treatment at a hospital. Providers use algorithms to determine when and how much medication to administer for a safe and optimal outcome. A key component of this assessment is determining the severity of alcohol withdrawal using the Clinical Institute Withdrawal Assessment for Alcohol (CIWA-Ar). The scale contains 10 subjective and objective items that can be queried and scored in minutes. Symptoms asked about include nausea, vomiting, tremors, sweating, anxiety, agitation, tactile/auditory/visual disturbances, headache, and cognitive dysfunction. Every hospital has different cutoffs for treatment, but as a general rule, treatment with benzodiazepines begin starting at a score 8–10, with higher scoring indicating increasing amount and frequency of medication.

---

5.   The memo is advising staff dealing with agitated patients on how to

    (**A**)   identify the cause of the agitation.

    (**B**)   avoid adding to the feelings of agitation.

    (**C**)   deal with violent behaviour caused by the agitation.

For the attention of all staff:

RE: AGITATED PATIENTS

Agitated patients are a common occurrence in the Emergency Department. There are many reasons for agitation, ranging from medical conditions, substance intoxication, psychiatric illness, and distressing circumstances. While both physical and chemical restraints are available to providers, these are items of last resort as their use creates significant risk to the patient, staff, and other persons in the area. Verbal de-escalation is a proven, effective technique that can be used to calm a patient down and promote a safe treatment environment. When de-escalating, designate one person to speak for the group. Agitated patients can be easily confused by multiple speakers and a unified message must be presented. Respect personal space to prevent the patient from feeling 'trapped' and maintain sufficient distance to avoid any resultant physical aggression. Remember to introduce yourself and your role on the treatment team to the patient. Use their name and orient them to their surroundings and why they are here in the hospital.

---

6.   The guidelines advise that patients with heart problems

(A)   may need to avoid ibuprofen.

(B)   should be given lidocaine for pain relief.

(C)   must receive a lower dose of acetaminophen.

EXTRACT FROM APPROPRIATE TREATMENT FOR PAIN

Pain is one of the most common complaints that will be brought to a physician's attention. This section will cover treatment of mild to moderate pain without the use of opioids. More severe pain may require judicious use of short-acting opioid medications or a consult to pain medicine. For most patients, the first line medications for pain are acetaminophen and ibuprofen. Maximum daily dosage of acetaminophen is suggested to be 4 grams, reduced to under 2 grams for patients with liver issues such as a cirrhosis. Ibuprofen is particularly effective in patients whose pain is caused by inflammation, though caution is urged in elderly patients, patients with diagnosed bleeding issues (especially gastrointestinal bleeds), or any cardiac issues. Maximum daily dosage suggested is 2.4 grams. A combination of acetaminophen and ibuprofen can be used if either one used alone is not sufficient. For more localised pain relief, consider using lidocaine dermal patches over non-broken areas of skin.

Answers

1	A	duty to care for a patient continues after a referral.
2	C	should only be used on patients as a last resort.
3	A	seeking advice from others.
4	C	They must be destroyed after use.
5	B	prevent a scab from forming.
6	C	who have a particular genetic makeup.
7	A	are caused by surgery.
8	C	what to do before administering an IV.
9	B	aware that even minor illnesses can be distressing for parents.
10	C	Inform patients of the changes to be implemented.

Practice Set

1	B	to prolong the effects
2	B	collect information about patients from their friends and relatives.
3	C	identify the cause through physical examination and tests.
4	A	determining the quantity of medication required.
5	C	deal with violent behaviour caused by the agitation.
6	A	may need to avoid ibuprofen.

CHAPTER 8

Reading Part C

LEARNING OBJECTIVES

By the end of this chapter, you will be able to:

- Briefly look through the text to understand the general meaning.
- Look for cues and prompts in the question to find the relevant information in the text.
- Identify the main idea of a text and of each paragraph.
- Practise strategies for answering Detail, Attitude and Opinion, Vocabulary and Reference questions.

Introduction

In Part C of the Reading Test, there are two texts, with eight questions on each one. The type of texts you will encounter will be in the style of articles published for a healthcare audience in a healthcare setting. They will not be specifically aimed at any one healthcare profession, and will use terminology that can be understood by any healthcare professional.

There is a combined time of 45 minutes for Parts B and C. If you spent roughly 10 minutes to complete Part B of the Reading Test, you will have 35 minutes to complete Part C of the test.

Strategies

Know the Instructions

You should make sure you are familiar with what you will be asked to do before you take the test. The instructions for Part C of the Reading Test will look like this:

In this part of the test, there are two texts about different aspects of healthcare. For **questions 7 to 22**, choose the answer (**A**, **B**, **C** or **D**) which you think fits best according to the text.

Write your answers on the separate **Answer Sheet**.

Know the Format

Each question refers to a discrete part of the text, and the questions appear in the order of the information in the text. You need to answer 8 questions on each of the 2 texts in this section of the test. The questions will direct you to the part of the text which the question refers, so you don't need to skim the entire text to find the information. In addition, once you have answered a question about one part of the text, you only need to look at the information that follows for the remaining questions, you will not need to look at the previous information.

Look at the Text

The first thing you should do, when tackling a Part C text, is to quickly look through the text, to understand how the text is organised and what it's about. As you skim through the text, you might find it helpful to make a few brief notes about the main idea or topic of each paragraph, to help you to remember what the text discusses. Don't worry about understanding the text in detail at this point, just give yourself a general sense of the text. When you come to answer the questions, the questions will guide you through the text.

Exercise

Take 5 minutes to skim-read the text below. As you look through, make brief notes about the content – aim for just 4 or 5 words or phrases per paragraph. Time yourself.

Text 1: Synthetic Voices

There are many reasons why a patient may lose their voice; indeed, many of us will already have experienced partial loss of voice, when suffering from a cold or flu. While we tend to dismiss a hoarse voice as a mild annoyance, when permanent voice loss occurs, it can be tremendously difficult for the patient to deal with, both practically, and emotionally. When our voice works, we don't spend too much time thinking about what life would be like without it, but the truth is that our voice is an integral part of who we are. Our voices define us, they allow our loved ones to identify us over the phone, or when visibility is poor. They distinguish us as individuals from certain parts of the world, and they can even indicate our social standing. Until recently, patients who experienced permanent loss of voice would have had relatively few options at their disposal. However, as technology advances, the range of speech replacement options available becomes increasingly sophisticated.

Today, synthetic voices are the most common type of speech replacement device used by those who have permanently lost their voice. The technology used to create this software can also be seen in speech controlled home devices, and modern smartphones. As permanent loss of voice is often caused by respiratory issues resulting from other illnesses, however, it's important that speech replacement devices for those who have lost their voice take the patient's other disabilities into account. Speech-to-text systems typically involve a system of levers or a simplified keyboard; the latter tends to be easier for those with limited mobility to operate. Users are able to manipulate these controls in order to select words from a computer interface and build them into sentences. Some systems can also operate via eye movement alone, so that when a user stares at a particular word on the screen for a certain amount of time, it is selected.

These systems show a remarkable advancement from one of the earliest speech-to-text mechanisms designed in the sixties: a typewriter operated through an air pipe, known as a sip and puff typewriter. The first electrical communication device for disabled people who could not speak, a sip and puff typewriter called the POSM (Patient Oriented Selector Mechanism), was developed by Reg Maling, a volunteer at a hospital for paralysed people, after he discovered that patients at the hospital who had lost the use of their voice were only able to communicate using a bell. Throughout the rest of the twentieth century, these technologies were gradually developed, and in the 1970s, the first portable, commercially available, adaptive alternative communication devices (or AACs), were produced. Although they were advertised as portable, these devices often weighed a hefty 15 – 20 pounds, and tended to range from 20 to 25 inches in size. As many of the early portable AAC users also used a wheelchair, in which it was relatively straightforward to design a holster at the back of the chair to store these devices.

Thankfully, the technology continued to develop, and devices became smaller, easier to use and more sophisticated. In the United States there are now over two million people who rely on such devices in their day-to-day communications, yet many users still have to make do with a limited number of vocal choices—often less than a dozen, with the majority of available voices sounding adult and/or male. This is extremely problematic, as users need to choose a voice that they feel represents who they are. Proponents of new digital voice banks are working toward **raising the bar** by steadily widening the scope for self-expression among the many millions of diverse users of AACs.

If patients are gradually losing their voice, but still able to speak, they may be able to record their own voice to use with their AAC. Another alternative open to patients is to make use of the increasing number of voices being donated. Although voice donation does not require the contributor to physically give a part of themselves away, as is the case with classic medical donations, donators certainly must **go the extra mile**. The process of voice donation is much more extensive than, say, donating a kidney, or other physical organ. While the donation of an organ requires a relatively short stay in hospital, to donate a voice requires many weeks of donor commitment. Donors must speak many thousands of preselected words, phrases and sentences into a recording microphone. Some companies offer a service tailored to the **user**, who can read science fiction or fantasy stories out loud—or texts according to their interests—in order to remain more engaged in the process.

Once a voice has been comprehensively recorded, it then becomes part of the software for AACs, and made available to any patient that needs it. Professor Stephen Hawking, the famous Cambridge physicist, began to use an early text-to-speech system in 1986 called CallText. Interestingly, the professor never changed his synthetic voice to a more sophisticated design that better imitated natural speech. Instead, Hawking retained CallText, explaining that he felt the limited modulations of the voice allowed his speech to be easier to hear and understand during lectures. Clearly, Hawking also came to see **it** as a part of his identity. 30 years after he began using CallText, the software was nearing breakdown, but rather than simply replace it, he had a team of researchers reverse engineer the voice onto a more modern platform.

Answer the Different Question Types

Once you've scanned the text, you can begin to work through the 8 questions. You should aim to spend one to one and a half minutes answering each question in this section, so make sure to time yourself accurately as you complete the exercises in this chapter.

When you come to answer the questions in Part C, first look at what the question is asking you to do, then scan the relevant paragraph of information, then look at the answer options. Mark any answer options that definitely do not answer the question with a cross, and if you're stuck between two answer choices, read through the relevant information again, then if you still can't find the answer, select one of the answer choices as a guess and move on.

The questions in Part C of the Reading Test can be broadly divided into 3 different question types. We will go through each question type below, and provide examples for each question type.

Detail, Attitude and Opinion

Detail, Attitude and Opinion questions will ask you to identify information from a section of a text, and will most often focus on the views and opinions of the writer. These questions are the most common question type in Part C. The following list gives examples of the types of Detail, Attitude and Opinion questions that occur in this section:

> *What point does the writer make in the third paragraph?*
>
> *The writer suggests that macular degeneration may increase*
>
> *In the fourth paragraph, the writer says that conventional treatments can be problematic because*

IMPROVE YOUR SCORE

Questions in Part C of the Reading Test always appear in text order and will often direct you to the relevant paragraph. Once you've answered a question about one part of the text, move on to the next part.

Exercise

Take 5 minutes to answer questions **1 – 4**. Time yourself.

1.   In the first paragraph, the writer suggests loss of voice is difficult for patients because it is

   (A)   part of their identity.

   (B)   necessary for interaction.

   (C)   used to form relationships.

   (D)   an indicator of social class.

2.   Why does the writer believe it is important that speech replacement devices be operated by a variety of methods?

   (A)   The technology should be kept up to date.

   (B)   Patients often suffer from various conditions.

   (C)   Healthcare workers might also need to use them.

   (D)   The devices should be usable across a range of platforms.

3.   In the third paragraph, we lean that Reg Malling developed the POSM due to

   (A)   the number of people who had permanently lost their voice.

   (B)   the lack of accessibility in previous sip and puff designs.

   (C)   the limited communication options for disabled people.

   (D)   the recent development of similar sound technology.

4.   According to the writer, why were early portable AACs problematic for those not in wheelchairs?

   (A)   They were heavy and bulky.

   (B)   They were remarkably fragile.

   (C)   They could not be used while walking.

   (D)   They needed access to a power source.

IMPROVE YOUR SCORE

Wrong answer choices will often feature other details from the text that are not asked about in the question, or will not reflect the meaning of the text. Make sure you are picking the detail that answers the question being asked.

Vocabulary

Vocabulary questions will present you with a single word or phrase that will be underlined and formatted in bold in the question and the text. To answer these questions correctly, you will need to look at the surrounding words and deduce the meaning added by the word or phrase. These questions are not testing your knowledge of the definition of the word or phrase itself. You should expect to answer one Vocabulary question in each text in Part C. The following list gives examples of Vocabulary questions:

*The writer uses the phrase '**cut corners**' to reinforce the idea that*

*In the final paragraph, the writer uses the phrase '**in the loop**' to underline*

*What is suggested about the attitude towards the trial by the use of the phrase '**on the fence**'?*

Exercise

Take 2 minutes and 30 seconds to answer questions **5 – 6**. Time yourself.

5.   The writer uses the phrase '**raising the bar**' to underline the

    (A) complexity of modern devices.

    (B) need for a diverse range of voices.

    (C) high quality of the sound recordings.

    (D) number of new communication systems.

6.   What is suggested about voice donation by the phrase '**go the extra mile**'?

    (A) donation centres are often far away

    (B) a large number of voices are rejected

    (C) donators sacrifice more than organ donators

    (D) the process is extremely time-consuming

Reference

Reference questions will ask you to decide what the word or phrase underlined and in bold in the question and in the text relates to. To answer these questions, you might need to be able to keep track of what is being discussed in long sections of text with complex sentences. You should expect to answer one Reference question in each passage in Part C. The following list gives examples of Reference questions:

*In the second paragraph, what does the word '**it**' refer to?*

*What does the word '**they**' refer to?*

*The phrase '**because of this**' refers to*

Exercise

Take 2 minutes and 30 seconds to answer questions **7 – 8**. Time yourself.

7.   In the fifth paragraph, the word '**user**' refers to

   (A)   healthcare workers who treat loss of voice.

   (B)   patients with permanent loss of voice.

   (C)   AAC technology developers.

   (D)   voice donators.

8.   What does the word '**it**' refer to in the final paragraph?

   (A)   A presentation given by the professor.

   (B)   The research carried out for the professor.

   (C)   The synthetic voice used by the professor.

   (D)   The permanent loss of voice of the professor.

IMPROVE YOUR SCORE

Practise for Part C of the Reading Test by reading newspaper articles, papers and studies written in English on healthcare topics. Pick an article with around 800 words and give yourself 5 minutes to read the text and make notes on the content.

Part C of the Reading Test is designed to evaluate your ability to quickly read and understand English texts in a healthcare setting. Make reading healthcare texts in English a habit to prepare yourself for the test. On Test Day, take a deep breath, read each section carefully, select an answer, then move on to the next question.

IMPROVE YOUR SCORE

Whenever you read articles, papers or studies in English, make a list of any words you do not recognise. Be sure to look up the meaning of each word, and note a synonym or non-technical term for this word. Building your vocabulary, and your confidence with unfamiliar words will boost your performance on Test Day.

Reading Part C Practice Set

For **questions 1 to 16**, choose the answer (**A**, **B**, **C** or **D**) which you think fits best according to the text.

Write your answers on the separate **Answer Sheet**.

Text 1: Delivering Serious News

Delivering serious news to patients and relatives: it's many healthcare professionals' most dreaded task. Unfortunately, it's not something that can be avoided, and it's something that must be done right. Patients and relatives need our guidance and support, particularly when the prognosis is serious. In this article, we use the phrase 'serious news' or 'life-altering news' rather than choosing a term with negative connotations, such as 'bad news', for example, as it helps to reframe the discussion. If you discuss 'serious news' with a patient, they can decide how to respond, whereas giving a patient 'bad news', may prevent them from being able to accept the news in a more constructive light.

Studies show the vast majority of patients would prefer to be informed of a life-altering diagnosis, rather than remain in ignorance. However, the amount of information they wish to receive can vary, with most wanting to know details concerning the different treatment options, and the effectiveness of proposed treatments, while they may want to hear less about the specific details of their prognosis. According to statistics, in western cultures, the majority of patients may not wish to know certain details, such as life expectancy. Healthcare workers may also find families asking that diagnoses be kept from the patient, or that patients prefer to have care wholly managed by their family, rather than themselves.

One model for delivering serious news is called SPIKES, developed by Walter Baile and initially used for discussions with cancer patients. The first step in SPIKES is setting up the interview. A quiet private area such as an exam room or family meeting room is an ideal setting. The patient should be able to choose family members or friends to be present for support. For **those** who don't speak fluent English, a hospital-contracted medical interpreter should be used. The healthcare professional should be prepared to answer difficult queries about prognosis, treatment, and overall plan going forward, but also know when to refer to a specialist for more esoteric information. If there is a multi-disciplinary approach, every team member should be on the same page with regards to the care plan to avoid confusion.

The second item in SPIKES is the patient's perception. Last week, I asked a patient, let's call him Harry, if he understood his current condition. Of course, he said he did, but when he came to explain it to me, I saw that there were many gaps in his knowledge that needed to be addressed. A good way to assess the patient's understanding is to ask what the patient already knows about their condition and what they have been told so far. Make sure to assess the level of their understanding, as well as their awareness of the basic facts. This will allow you to assess their level of background knowledge, their current knowledge, and where to begin your own discussion.

The third item in SPIKES is the patient's invitation for discussion. Different patients desire different levels of information about their condition. Some of the more technical-minded or younger patients may want to know their diagnosis, prognosis, treatments, course of illness, etc. Others, including older patients, may simply wish to know the diagnosis and accept the recommendations of the treatment team as being in their best interests. Before beginning to discuss their condition, you might find it helpful to ask "Would you like me to discuss all the information we know about your condition or just certain parts? What would you like us to tell your family?"

The fourth item in SPIKES is giving knowledge to the patient. You should be direct, but avoid being unfeeling or blunt when you discuss their condition, and utilise non-technical terms in small chunks. Prognosis and course of illness should be realistic, but also convey hope and planning for the future. An appropriate opening for our patient would be, "I'm afraid, we have some serious news about the CT scan that was performed. It showed that the cancer in your liver has spread to your spine." Take note of how the words 'hepatocellular carcinoma' and 'metastasis' were rephrased into layman's terms.

The fifth item in SPIKES is addressing the patient's emotions. You should identify the emotion the patient is experiencing, the reasoning, and provide support during this difficult time. Don't try to change the patient's emotions, just help them to express how they feel. For example, in a patient who is dysphoric and crying, you can offer a tissue box and physical support if appropriate. You might say something like, "I know these results weren't what you wanted to hear. I wish we had better news for you." Other responses can range from asking the patient to elaborate on their reaction, "Can you tell me what you're worried about?" to validating their concerns, "I can understand why you felt that way. Many other patients have had similar reactions."

The sixth item in SPIKES is strategy and summary. Patients who receive serious news will often feel that they are **in over their head**, so you should make sure that they leave with a clear plan for the future. This will help them to feel less anxious and more hopeful. Patients should know what options are available for them and what follow-up is planned. You should also recheck that they understand what has just been discussed and have had all their questions answered. A good opening statement could be, "I understand this is a lot to take in, but you have several options available. A decision does not need to be made now, but we would like to refer you to an oncologist and follow-up with us in a week to discuss your next steps."

Giving serious news is one of the most difficult parts of being a healthcare professional. However, with careful planning and an effective protocol, patients can leave feeling well-informed and in control of their own outcome.

Text 1: Questions 1 to 8

1.   Why does the writer prefer the term 'serious news'?

   (A) It enables doctors to avoid unnecessary conversations.

   (B) It avoids influencing the patient's emotional response.

   (C) It helps patients to better understand their condition.

   (D) It offers a more specific definition of the information.

2.   The writer's purpose in the second paragraph is to highlight

   (A) the treatment options available to most patients.

   (B) the difficulty of knowing what a patient wants to be told.

   (C) the trends concerning what patients and relatives want to hear.

   (D) the different topics that healthcare workers should cover with patients.

3.   What does the word **'those'** refer to?

   (A) healthcare staff

   (B) treatment experts

   (C) language translators

   (D) patients and relatives

4.   In the fourth paragraph, the writer mentions the patient, Harry, in order to explain that

   (A) patients are often reluctant to ask for help.

   (B) patients may not be aware of their ignorance.

   (C) healthcare professionals often find it hard to relate to patients.

   (D) healthcare professionals may not always explain things effectively.

5.   The writer suggests that older patients may be more likely to

   (A) require more information.

   (B) limit their family's involvement.

   (C) accept the staff's suggested plan.

   (D) inquire further about their treatment plans.

6.   In the sixth paragraph, the writer offers an example to emphasise that when explaining information professionals should

   (A) avoid using complex medical language.

   (B) prevent patients from becoming upset.

   (C) discuss how the illness was identified.

   (D) repeat information multiple times.

7. The seventh paragraph focuses on

   (A) ensuring the patient understands how to react.

   (B) helping the patient to feel more positive.

   (C) comparing different patient responses.

   (D) empathising with the patient's reaction.

8. The expression **'in over their head'** is used to stress that patients might

   (A) find the information overwhelming.

   (B) struggle to remember information.

   (C) make a choice about their treatment quickly.

   (D) have difficulty understanding their prognosis.

In this part of the test, there are two texts about different aspects of healthcare. For **questions 9 to 16**, choose the answer (**A**, **B**, **C** or **D**) which you think fits best according to the text.

Write your answers on the separate **Answer Sheet**.

Text 2: Treating Opium Addiction

In the United States alone, there are around 115 deaths caused by opioid addiction every day. The addiction impacts individuals rapidly and drastically, damages families, and costs the US huge amounts of money: the total economic burden of prescription opioid abuse is estimated to be $78.5 billion a year, while the economic burden of non-prescription opioid abuse simply cannot be calculated. Measures are constantly being improved to prevent patients from developing opioid addictions to begin with, but it is also imperative that we continue to provide treatment for those already in the thrall of opioid addiction.

Jane's story is one heard over and over again in opioid addiction clinics. When she was 20, she had a bad automobile accident that required two surgeries. She was soon home from the hospital but her residual pain meant she was prescribed scheduled opiates. Jane's body soon became tolerant of the dosage; however, and she needed higher and higher doses in order to achieve the same pain relieving effect. She eventually reached a level that her physician felt uncomfortable prescribing. Unable to find another prescriber in time, Jane turned to alternative sources of narcotics. Unfortunately, when purchased on the street, these pills are exorbitantly expensive and increasingly hard to come by in an era of prescription monitoring throughout the United States. Heroin is much cheaper and, when delivered by IV, produces a much more potent high and greater pain relief.

Eventually, after destroying relationships with her loved ones, bankrupting her savings, and **hitting rock-bottom**, Jane turned to a local opioid addiction clinic for help. At the clinic, they put her on Methadone, a long-acting opioid agonist that is standard for addiction treatment. It binds to the mu-opioid receptors, prevents withdrawal symptoms, reduces cravings, and can also provide a level of pain relief. Of course, as an opioid agonist, methadone serves as a substitute for the primary addiction, meaning many of the issues associated with long-term opioid usage remain. Patients must often begin treatment with daily visits, which can be disruptive. Fortunately for Jane, these visits are her first steps towards putting her life back together. As Jane's road to recovery is likely to be long and fraught with difficulty, many doctors are led to wonder: does she have any other options?

One of the increasingly popular alternatives to methadone is buprenorphine, a partial mu-opioid agonist. Aside from its unique mechanism of action (MOA), there are two major differences when compared to Methadone: first, it can be administered as oral tablets, sublingual/buccal films, and a long-acting implant, second, It can be prescribed month-to-month from a clinician's office directly to a local pharmacy. These factors make it much easier to use in the community, and are ideal for patients who cannot visit a methadone clinic every day.

To initiate buprenorphine, a patient must already be in a mild state of withdrawal due to the high affinity for the mu-opioid receptor displacing other opioids. **This means that** patients generally transition best from a short-acting opioid like heroin or oxycodone rather than a long-acting opioid agonist like Methadone, given the length of time needed until mild withdrawal occurs. As Jane had been using opioids for a long time prior to her admission, however, she was better suited to treatment with Methadone, as there is no ceiling effect to this drug, and Jane had developed a high tolerance to opioids. Buprenorphine, being a partial agonist, has a maximum level of effect which it cannot be increased beyond. For this reason, buprenorphine can be used as a maintenance therapy in some patients, but it can also be tapered down over time. This allows patients to resume their normal lives with minimal interruptions and avoid relapse through pharmacological blocking.

Alongside treatment with medication, patients recovering from opioid addiction must also deal with recovery at a mental level. As with many healing processes, the first stage is acceptance. Jane was not able to seek the treatment she needed until she had nowhere else to hide. Once everything was lost, she couldn't deny that she was in trouble anymore, so she came to the clinic. Many patients suffering from opioid addictions are reluctant to admit that they are addicted, and reluctant to ask for help. Patients are often worried about being judged, being treated like a criminal, and meeting with disapproval from the healthcare professionals who must treat them.

When patients do seek aid, healthcare professionals need to help them to build a support network around themselves, so that they are protected when they feel the need to relapse. Opioid addicts are likely to have burned bridges with friends and family who have not enabled their addiction, so patients beginning recovery may not have positive role models to support and influence their recovery. Talking therapies, such as cognitive behavioural therapy (CBT) can be offered to recovering patients experiencing anxiety or depression, though patients may find it more useful to join local confidential support groups, such as Narcotics Anonymous, as they can discuss recovery with those who have first-hand experience. Though Jane was hesitant to discuss her experiences with anyone when she was first admitted to the clinic for treatment, she has since gone on to attend weekly sessions at Narcotics Anonymous, where she not only listens to others share their stories of recovery, but where she also is beginning to tell her own.

Text 1: Questions 9 to 16

9. In the first paragraph, the writer highlights that opioid addiction in the US

    (A) has been gradually increasing for a number of years.

    (B) is largely influenced by the illegal sale of drugs.

    (C) causes more deaths than any other addiction.

    (D) has a significant financial and social impact.

10. In the second paragraph, the writer outlines Jane's case in order to emphasise that

    (A) opioid addiction is increasingly rare.

    (B) it can be remarkably easy for a patient to become addicted.

    (C) in some cases, heroin is less harmful to addicts than opioids.

    (D) healthcare professionals must take responsibility for opioid addiction.

11. The writer uses the phrase '**hitting rock bottom**' about the patient Jane in order to describe

    (A) how her addiction led to the most distressing point in her life.

    (B) her sudden awareness that she had to recover.

    (C) the large tolerance she developed for opioids.

    (D) the physical pain she felt at that time.

12. In the fourth paragraph, the writer suggests that buprenorphine may be preferable because

    (A) it is less addictive than alternatives.

    (B) it can be easier for patients to access.

    (C) it does not interfere with other treatments.

    (D) it can be picked up more often than other medications.

13. What does '**this means that**' refer to?

    (A) The effectiveness of buprenorphine when combating opioid displacement.

    (B) The requirement for the medication to be reserved for heroin addicts.

    (C) The need for patients to have begun to experience withdrawals.

    (D) The impact of mu-opioids on recovered opioid addicts.

14. In the fifth paragraph, the writer suggests that Jane was prescribed methadone, rather than buprenorphine because

    (A) buprenorphine is too similar to heroin.

    (B) the effects of methadone last for longer.

    (C) she was dependent on high doses of opioids.

    (D) it is more readily available at addiction clinics.

15. According to the seventh paragraph, why do patients often delay seeking treatment for opioid addiction?

    (A) They are unwilling to face the damage they have caused.

    (B) They do not realise they are addicted until it's too late.

    (C) They think that they can recover without help.

    (D) They do not want to be labelled as an addict.

16. In the final paragraph, the writer suggests that recovering addicts may prefer to discuss their experiences with

    (A) those who have experienced addiction.

    (B) people who are not aware of their history.

    (C) healthcare professionals.

    (D) friends and family.

Answers

1	A	part of their identity.
2	B	patients often suffer from various conditions.
3	C	The limited communication options for disabled people.
4	A	They were heavy and bulky.
5	B	need for a diverse range of voices.
6	D	the process is extremely time-consuming.
7	D	voice donators.
8	C	The synthetic voice used by the professor.

Practice Sets

Questions 1 to 8

1	B	It avoids influencing the patient's emotional response.
2	C	the trends concerning what patients and relatives want to hear.
3	D	patients and relatives
4	B	patients may not be aware of their ignorance.
5	C	accept the staff's suggested plan.
6	A	avoid using complex medical language.
7	D	empathising with the patient's reaction.
8	A	find the information overwhelming.

Questions 9 to 16

9	D	has a significant financial and social impact.
10	B	it can be remarkably easy for a patient to become addicted.
11	A	how her addiction led to the most distressing point in her life.
12	B	it can be easier for patients to access.
13	C	The need for patients to have begun to experience withdrawals.
14	C	she was dependent on high doses of opioids.
15	D	They do not want to be labelled as an addict.
16	A	those who have experienced addiction.

PART FOUR

The Writing Section

Writing Introduction

Section Overview

The Writing Test in OET consists of one task, which you must complete in 40 minutes after being allowed 5 minutes of reading time. You must read the notes provided about a patient and their treatment, then write a letter of between 180 and 200 words approximately to a person named in the task. You will be provided with a letter writing task, which will tell you what sort of letter to write, who to write to, and several pages of patient's case notes, which you will write about in your letter.

The writing task will be specific to your healthcare profession. In this book, we will cover writing tasks for those working in Medical and Nursing professions.

The letter you write should use information from the patient notes to complete the task effectively, and be within the word limit.

Writing Strategies

- Know the instructions and format before Test Day, so you know what to expect ahead of the test: you will always be asked to write a letter of 180 to 200 words, and you will always be given patient case notes.
- Start by reading the writing task section at the end of the test to find out what sort of letter you need to write, and who to write the letter to.
- Read through the case notes, starting with who you are in relation to the patient.
- Continue reading through the case notes, thinking about what's relevant to your letter as you do so. Please note that you are unable to underline key words or phrases during the 5 minutes' reading time.
- Plan your letter by outlining what you will include in response to the writing task.
- Keep your plan brief and write in note form.
- Write your letter, using information in the patient case notes where necessary.
- Do not write additional patient information into your letter which is not contained in the case notes, you must not make up patient history, or propose treatment options if they are not given in the notes.
- Do not include any information from the patient case notes that is not relevant to the letter requirements.

- Make sure the tone of your writing is appropriate. If you're writing to another health-care professional, you should use medical terminology where relevant. If you're writing to a layperson, such terminology should be avoided. The tone of the letter should always be formal.

- Where possible, use a range of tenses, grammar and vocabulary to demonstrate your writing skills.

- Aim to complete your letter at least 3 minutes before the end of the test, so that you have time to read through your letter and correct any mistakes.

CHAPTER 9

The Writing Task

LEARNING OBJECTIVES

By the end of this chapter, you will be able to:

- Analyse the task.
- Scan the patient case notes for relevant information.
- Plan your letter effectively.
- Practise writing a letter within the word and time limits.

Introduction

In the OET Writing Test, you will be asked to write one letter to another person involved in a patient's care. You will have 40 minutes to plan, write and review your letter, with an additional 5 minutes at the start to read the letter writing task and patient case notes.

The Writing Test will be specific to your healthcare profession. In this chapter, we will look at examples for Nursing and Medicine.

The Writing Test is assessed using 5 criteria. To get a good mark in this section of the test, you must score well in each section. Below is an overview of the marking criteria used by OET assessors to grade the writing tasks, we will go into more detail about how to score well in each section later on in this chapter.

Overall task fulfilment

You must complete the task with an appropriate response that accurately addresses the writing task and is roughly within the word count. For example, the letter should be between 180 and 200 words, and if the task asks you to write a letter of discharge, you must make sure that the letter actually states that the patient is being discharged.

Appropriateness of language

You must make sure the tone of your letter is appropriate to the task, and the register (level of formality and technicality) is suitable for the situation. If the writing task asks you to write to another healthcare professional, it is appropriate to use medical language, while if the task asks you to write to a layperson, you might use more everyday language, and explain technical words. This criteria also takes into account the organisation of the letter, with appropriate sequencing of the information appropriate to the genre.

Comprehension of stimulus

You must write a letter for the task that uses the necessary information from the case notes, and does not use unnecessary points. This criterion tests your ability to understand the writing task and the patient's notes. To achieve a good score, you should make sure you use all of the information that is relevant to the task in the case notes for your letter, and only the relevant information. For example, it is unlikely that you would need to include information about the patient's history of illness if you are writing a letter to their GP or family doctor.

Control of linguistic features

You must use correct grammar in your letter, show a range of grammatical structures and write a letter that is cohesive and follows a logical order. Make sure to read through your letter after you have finished writing it, to look for any errors in your writing, so that you can fix these before you finish your test.

Control of presentation features

You must avoid spelling errors, use correct punctuation, and use clear letter layout.

Strategies

Begin with the letter writing task

Before you start to look at the information in the patient case notes, you should first turn to look at the letter writing task. This will inform you of the task, including who you need to write to, and what you need to say. You should aim to spend 30 seconds looking at the writing task to determine what information is important, the reason that you are writing the letter, and to think about what your response will include, before moving on to the next stage.

Exercise

Take 30 seconds to look at the writing task below, then answer questions **1 – 5** that follow.

Writing Task

Using the information given in the case notes, write a letter of referral for Mr Walter Peters to Dr N Shah, the Admitting Officer at New Canterbury Hospital, 1 Church Street, Canterbury, for further assessment and treatment.

In your answer:

- **Expand the relevant notes into complete sentences**
- **Do not use note form**
- **Use letter format**

The body of the letter should be approximately 180 – 200 words.

1. Who is the patient?
2. Who will the letter be addressed to?
3. What is happening, that must be described in the letter?
4. Where must the letter be addressed?

The section of the writing task shown in bold will be the same for every writing task, so make sure you are familiar with these instructions. The instructions emphasise the importance of taking the case notes and altering them where possible, to create a letter that not only communicates the task given in the letter writing task, but does so in a way that demonstrates your writing abilities. To get a high score, you must expand the case notes, and create a letter that uses complex sentences, a range of appropriate vocabulary, and various grammatical structures.

The case notes you will be provided with will be written in brief note form. The case notes will often include short words and phrases which are not complete sentences, and they may include commonly used medical abbreviations. The case notes have been written by a healthcare professional, for other healthcare professionals within their hospital or clinic, so a certain amount of understanding is expected. As such, as well as expanding the case notes into full sentences, you should also make sure that you change the wording so that it is suitable for the intended audience, given in the task. While you read the task, you should begin to consider how you might demonstrate your writing skills in this task and respond appropriately to the task.

The writing task will usually ask you to write a letter of referral. Other types of letter which might be used in the test include a discharge letter or a letter of explanation.

Scan the Case Notes Actively

The next stage in the writing task is to scan the patient case notes, while keeping the letter writing task in mind. The patient case notes provided will cover several pages, and provide a lot of information. You are not allowed to underline words or write on the case notes during this time, but you should scan the case notes actively, and identify keywords, phrases and information that are relevant to the letter you will need to write, so that you can incorporate them into your letter. You should spend the whole 5 minutes reading time scanning the patient case notes carefully, and identifying relevant information.

Exercise

Scan the patient case notes below, and make a mental note of any key pieces of information that would be relevant for a letter writing task that asked you to write a letter of discharge to a rehab facility. Time yourself for 5 minutes and after this time has elapsed, go through the case notes, underlining anything which you thought to be relevant.

Notes:

Ms Lydia Frank is a 49-year-old female who was transferred from the neuro intensive care unit (NICU) to the neuro telemetry unit.

Hospital:	Lexington Hospital
Patient details	
Name:	Lydia Frank
Marital status:	Divorced for 8 years
Next of kin:	Darlene (daughter – 24-years-old, unemployed)
Admission date:	20 January 2018
Discharge date:	13 April 2018
Diagnosis:	Subarachnoid hemorrhage (SAH)

IMPROVE YOUR SCORE

Time yourself every time you write a practice letter. Always allow a few minutes before the time is up to check your work for spelling mistakes, inappropriate words and any other problems with your grammar or phrasing.

Past medical history:	Hypertension (2015)
	Hyperlipidemia
	Migraine
	Anxiety and depression
	Smoker (approx. 10 cigs per week)
Social background:	Works full time-accountant, financially independent.
Presenting Complaint:	Found unresponsive at work. Complaining of "worst headache ever". Admission 20/01/2018
Assessment:	Vomitus present. SAH. Pupils equal, round + reactive to light.
	BP 220/110 mm Hg. Endotracheal intubation performed (weaned from mechanical ventilation week 2).
	No supplemental oxygen required
	Craniotomy and endovascular coiling performed to treat SAH
	Developed central line-associated bloodstream infection and urinary tract infection – multiple rounds of IV antibiotics.
21/01/2018:	Oriented to person, place, time, and situation – slow to respond.
	BP very unstable.
	Antihypertensive medications adjusted 5 times since admission (currently taking clonidine PRN, scheduled lisinopril, scheduled labetalol).
	BP within normal limits (145/90-150/80 mm Hg – one week)
	No reports of headache 1/7. Left-sided weakness slowly improving.
Nursing management:	Neurologic and BP checks every 4 hours.
	Encourage patient to be seated in bedside chair for meals (→ requires 2 assists to pivot from bed to chair secondary to left-sided weakness). Requires assistance with feeding.
	Nectar thick liquids required.
	Medications crushed with apple sauce.
Assessment:	Good progress overall.
Discharge plan:	Discharge to rehab facility, continue nursing management as above.

Plan Your Response

During the reading time, read the letter writing task and identify relevant points to include in your letter from the case notes. You should now have an idea of what your letter will include. Once the writing time starts, the next stage is to plan your letter by outlining the structure of your correspondence. The keywords in the case notes are the words and phrases that relate to the purpose of the letter you need to write, for example, if you need to write a letter referring the patient for further assessment, then you should look for words in the case notes that relate to treatment. The information in the case notes that relates to past medical history is likely to include information that is not relevant to your letter.

Begin planning your letter by thinking about the person you are writing to. As mentioned earlier, think about the tone you will use for the person you are writing to, and also think about the information they will need to complete necessary actions after receiving your letter. Ask yourself the following questions as you plan:

1. Who are you writing to?
2. Why are you writing to them?
3. What do they need to know?
4. What do they know already?

The last question is important as in some cases, the person you are writing to will already be familiar with some of the information, so you should avoid using information from the case notes that they are already likely to know.

As you continue to plan your letter, think about where the different parts of information might appear. The case notes you are provided with will not necessarily present the information in the best order for your letter, so you should plan to use different areas of the case notes for various parts of your letter. It might be best to think about three or four broad points that you want to cover. For example, when writing a letter of discharge, you might want to discuss:

1. Why the patient was under your care.
2. How the patient was treated.
3. When the patient's current situation will change (if they are being discharged or referred).
4. What the patient's current state is, and what the patient's current treatment is.

Once you've decided on the points you will cover, you can begin to add to each point from the case notes. Remember that there are a variety of different approaches to the letter writing part of the test. The outline provided below offers an example of how you might structure your response to the task, but you may prefer to use a different outline to plan your letter. As you practise the writing task, try to vary your responses for each task, rather than following a set format. Practising different ways to write will improve your overall writing abilities, prepare you for an unexpected writing task on Test Day, and make sure you are prepared to write healthcare letters in English in the real world.

As an example, you might create the following plan for a letter of referral using the case notes about Lydia Frank on the previous two pages. Please note that you should avoid spending more than 5 minutes planning so you may not be able to develop such a detailed plan on Test Day.

Lydia Frank (F) to rehab facility

1. *Why was F admitted?*
   - *NICU 20 January 2018 – because subarachnoid hemorrhage (SAH) at work. unresponsive and receiving mechanical ventilation*

2. *What was treatment?*
   - *2nd week taken off mechanical ventilation - made good progress*
   - *at 1st - craniotomy + endovascular coiling – SAHMs. treatment complicated - central line-associated bloodstream infection + urinary tract infection*

3. *Current condition*
   - *F without infection good cough effort, no supplemental oxygen req., + aware of person, place, time, situation – BUT slow respond.*

4. *Current/future treatment?*
   - *F's blood pressure now controlled - scheduled lisinopril, scheduled labetalol, + PRN clonidine - crushed with apple sauce*
   - *nectar thick liquids a must*
   - *needs assistance 2 people - pivoting bed to chair + ambulation – left-sided weakness.*
   - *BP + neurological checks every 4 hours.*

Notice that the plan breaks the letter out into four separate sections, and uses information from the case notes to support each section.

Now, complete the exercise below using the case notes that begin below and finish on the following page, and the relevant Task 1 on page 130.

Exercise

Look at the writing task and patient case notes on the following pages. Take 5 minutes to read the case notes and identify the keywords, then take a further 5 minutes to make a brief plan for your letter.

Notes

Ms. Bethany Tailor is a 35-year-old patient in the psychiatric ward where you are working as a doctor or nurse.

Hospital:	St. Mary's Public Hospital, 32 Fredrick Street, Proudhurst
Patient Details:	Ms Bethany Tailor
	Next of Kin: Henry Tailor (father, 65) and Barbara Tailor (mother, 58)
Admission date:	01 March 2018
Discharge date:	18 March 2018

IMPROVE YOUR SCORE

Make sure you understand any case notes you will include in your letter, and make sure to put the patient case notes into your own words where possible, to achieve a high score on Test Day.

Diagnosis:	Schizophrenia
Past medical history:	Hypertension secondary to fibromuscular dysplasia
	Primary hypothyroidism Levothyroxine 88 mcg daily
Social background:	Unemployed, on disability allowance for schizophrenia.
	History of polysubstance abuse, mainly cocaine and alcohol.
	Last used cocaine 28/02/18
Admission 01/03/2018:	Patient self-admitted: decompensated schizophrenia
Medical background:	Not compliant with medications.
	Admitted for auditory command hallucinations telling patient to harm self.
	Visual hallucinations – shadow figures with grinning faces.
	Delusion – personal connections to various political leaders.
	01/03/2018 – agitated and aggressive, responding to internal stimuli with thought blocking and latency.
	Commenced antipsychotic meds (rispoderone).
	10/03/2018: Patient ceased reporting auditory or visual hallucinations.
	Less disorganised thinking. No signs of thought blocking or latency.
	Able to minimise delusions and focus on activities of daily living.
Nursing management:	Assess for objective signs of psychosis.
	Redirect patient from delusions.
	Ensure medical compliance.
	Help maintain behavioural control, provide therapy if possible.
Assessment:	Good progress, chronic mental illness, can decompensate if not on medications or abusing substances. Insight good, judgment fair.
Discharge plan:	Discharge on Risperidone 4g nightly by mouth.
	Risperidone 1 milligram available twice daily p.r.n for agitation or psychosis.
	Discharge back to apartment with follow-up at Proudhurst Mental Health Clinic.

Medical Writing Task 1

Using the information given in the case notes, write a discharge letter to the patient's primary care physician, Dr. Giovanni DiCoccio, Proudhurst Family Practice, 231 Brightfield Avenue, Proudhurst.

In your answer:

- **Expand the relevant notes into complete sentences**
- **Do not use note form**
- **Use letter format**

The body of the letter should be approximately 180 – 200 words.

Nursing Writing Task 1

Using the information given in the case notes, write a letter to the receiving nurse at the long-term care home where the patient will go following discharge, Maria DiCoccio, Proudhurst Mental Health Home, 231 Brightfield Avenue, Proudhurst.

In your answer:

- **Expand the relevant notes into complete sentences**
- **Do not use note form**
- **Use letter format**

The body of the letter should be approximately 180 – 200 words.

Write Your Letter

Once you've outlined the structure of your response, you can move on to writing the letter itself. Read through the following strategies to familiarise yourself with the type of letter you must write. The strategies will cover how you should write your letter, and the criteria you will be marked against.

Headings and Endings

Your letter should always begin by giving the date, the address and name or occupation of the person you're writing to, and a greeting to the person you're writing to. Below is an example of an appropriate introduction to a letter.

D J Horus

Perth Rehabilitation Hospital

23-40 Main Street

Perth

20 April 2018

Dear Dr Horus,

Exercise

5. Using the letter writing task provided on page 124, write an appropriate heading to a letter.

Practise following a similar format when you attempt your writing responses, until you are familiar with these headings.

Overall task fulfilment

To address this criteria, you should aim to write between 180–200 words in the body of your letter (after 'Dear___' and before 'Yours sincerely'). There is no need to count the exact number of words you have written but it is a good idea to know roughly how many lines of your handwriting are 180–200 words. You can work this out by counting the words of one full line of your writing and then dividing 200 by this number to give you the number of lines. Then, every time you complete a practise test, you can check you have roughly this number of lines.

If you have written more than this, check you have included all relevant information and left out all irrelevant information then edit accordingly. Keep in mind that your word count is just one indication that you've included relevant information. It's possible that you might have included the right information but still might fall slightly outside of the 180 to 200 word range. Falling outside of this word range does not necessarily mean you'll score poorly in this criteria.

You must also make sure that you are writing the type of letter specified in the task. Pay close attention to what this section says, and build your response around the task. Don't try to prepare a response before looking at the task, or try and memorise a letter that you can reproduce on Test Day, as this will not show that you are able to respond appropriately to the task that is given.

You should also avoid copying entire phrases exactly as they appear in the case notes. This is not a good plan for two reasons:

(1) The phrases used in the case notes are in note form. They are generally not appropriate in their current state for a letter, so you must expand these phrases, in order to write in an appropriate style.

(2) The assessor can also see the case notes. If you copy the language in the case notes exactly, the assessor will not be able to assess your understanding of the case notes, or your writing ability.

Demonstrate your skills by writing a letter that incorporates the relevant facts appropriately and in your own words.

IMPROVE YOUR SCORE

The more you practise writing within the word count, the easier it will become to predict how many words you need without counting. This will save valuable time on Test Day. To quickly estimate how many words you have used, you can count the number of words in one line of your letter, and then multiply this by the number of lines. However, as long as you make sure you are choosing all of the relevant case notes from the case study, and only the relevant case notes, your sample response should naturally fall within the word count.

Appropriateness of language

Letter tasks in the Writing Test will always ask you to write letters in the role of a healthcare professional. As such, you should always use a suitably formal tone in the writing section. You should avoid using casual language or idioms ('how's it going?'), and write in full words, rather than contractions ('can't' 'isn't') or SMS text abbreviations (use 'before', not 'b4').

If you are writing to a healthcare professional, you can use technical terminology, whereas, if you are writing to a layperson, you should make sure to explain medical terminology that may be unfamiliar.

You should always begin your letter by stating what the purpose of your letter is. If you're writing a letter of referral, you might begin your letter with a sentence like

> *Joanna Howards will be discharged to your Nursing Facility on 12 October 2018.*

Note that in this example we included the date, to make sure that the most important information is provided to the recipient of the letter in the first sentence. You should also include dates, times and time periods throughout your letter, and use language that clearly sequences the time-period of the information, in order to provide a clear order to your letter. For example, instead of writing

> *The patient was diagnosed with cancer of the oesophagus and had an oesophagectomy and chemotherapy and lost a considerable amount of weight.*

You could say something like this:

> *The patient was diagnosed with cancer of the oesophagus on 24th April. Chemotherapy was scheduled to begin in the following week and last for a total of three weeks. The patient lost a considerable amount of weight as a result of this treatment. An oesophagectomy was then successfully carried out on 3rd June.*

Look at the various ways the second example links the different pieces of information, and allows the reader to see the sequence of events more clearly.

If the task requires you to write an urgent letter, you should make this clear in your letter, too. An urgent letter may also require you to change the structure of the letter, for instance, you would need to put the patient's current condition at the beginning of an urgent letter, while if the letter was not urgent, it might be more appropriate to begin with the patient's history. The tone of your letter should always take into account your audience and the purpose of your letter. You can only use 180 – 200 words in your letter, so there is not enough room for you to include any unnecessary details.

Comprehension of stimulus

To meet this criterion, you need to show that you have understood the case notes. You can do this by using the case notes appropriately to create a letter that fully addresses the task.

Rather than trying to use as many case notes as possible, think about what the individual you are writing to needs to know. If you include information that is not relevant to the task, you will receive a lower score, so only include it if you think it is relevant to your letter. If you include too much surrounding detail, then it will also make it difficult for the assessor to assess that you have understood the task.

Put the case notes into your own words wherever possible, and connect the case notes together appropriately. Remember, you should not add any information to your letter that is not included in the case notes.

Exercise

Now that you've spent the 5 minutes reading time reading through the case notes, and another 5 minutes planning your response, spend another 35 minutes to complete your letter using the letter writing task and patient case notes on pages 128 – 130. Be sure to allow 3-5 minutes at the end to check your writing for errors.

_____

_____

_____

IMPROVE YOUR SCORE

Don't try to memorise long sections of letters to reproduce on Test Day. While it can be helpful to know general phrases and terminology to use in your letter, preparing larger sections of writing to use in your letter is unlikely to relate to the writing task, or make good use of the patient case notes, and will result in a lower writing score.

Check Your Letter for Errors

Once you have finished writing your letter, you should make sure to check through what you have written and correct any errors. Once you have looked through your letter and identified your errors, make a list of your most common errors, and make an effort to target these areas in particular, before completing another writing task. For example, if you commonly make article errors, make sure to revise the correct articles to use, for example, you should use 'in the bloodstream' rather than 'in bloodstream', and 'a heart attack' should be used, rather than 'an heart attack'.

Grammar and Cohesion

Make sure that you show that you can vary your language while writing the task. One way that you can show variation in your writing, is to talk about patient care in the past (for example, what has been done so far), the present (for example, the patient's current care plan) and the future (for example, how the patient's treatment should progress). You can use simple sentences, but you should also use complex sentences too. When you read through your letter, look at the length of the sentences you use. If you have lots of short sentences, consider using connectives to join some of these sentences into longer, complex sentences. On the other hand, if you have a lot of very long sentences, you might want to split this content up into smaller sentences, or remove information that is not necessary, to make sure that your writing is controlled.

Spelling and Punctuation

Your spelling and punctuation will also be assessed, so when you review your work you should make sure that your words are spelled correctly, and your punctuation is appropriate. In OET, you can use any spelling convention, such as American, Australian or British. Whichever spelling convention you choose to use, you must keep to this convention throughout your writing task. For your information, this book is written in British English.

When checking your work, if you spot a word that looks like it is spelled incorrectly, but you cannot remember how the word should be spelled, consider replacing it with a synonym that is easier for you to spell. It is more important that you communicate effectively than that you use long words. Remember that most of the healthcare terms you use will be in the case notes, so be sure to check your spelling of these words against the case notes as you review your letter.

Make sure that you are using enough full stops to separate distinct pieces of information, and using enough commas to separate your ideas within sentences. As you read through your work, read your letter to yourself in your head, pausing for commas and full stops, and check that it 'sounds' right to you. If it doesn't, look at changing your punctuation. Remember to leave space (one blank line is ideal) between each paragraph, so that the assessor can clearly see that you have sectioned your writing into a logical structure. Each paragraph should address one main point in your letter.

You need to write clearly and neatly, so that the assessor can easily read your handwriting. If your writing is difficult to read, the assessor may not be able to assess your writing ability. If you struggle with writing neatly and legibly, practise writing in English, and ask other people to read what you have written.

Exercise

After reading through the last two criteria in the section above, take 10 minutes to go over your letter and correct any mistakes.

Try to make reading and writing in English a part of your everyday life. The more you read, the better your writing will become. When you practise writing in English, you can focus on writing on more general topics, as well as focusing on healthcare topics. This will broaden your writing skills, and help you to score well on Test Day.

IMPROVE YOUR SCORE

Each time you write a practice letter, you should assess it based on the official OET criteria. Visit www.occupationalenglishtest.org to find the latest version. If possible, you could also ask a friend, family member or colleague with good English skills to assess your response.

Writing Practice Set

Read the case notes below and complete the Writing Tasks that follows. For each Writing Set, there are two Writing Tasks, one for Nursing, and one for Medicine. Choose the task that best reflects your healthcare profession. You should spend 5 minutes reading the case notes and 40 minutes writing your letter.

Notes:

You are a nurse OR a first year resident in a surgical ward. Sally Fletcher is a 25-year-old woman who has recently undergone surgery. You are now discharging her from hospital.

Hospital:	Fairbanks Hospital, 1001 Noble St, Fairbanks, AK 99701
Name:	Mrs Sally Fletcher
Date of Birth:	3/10/1993
Marital status:	Married, 5 years
Appointment date:	25/03/2018
Diagnosis:	Endometriosis
Past medical history:	Painful periods 3 years
	Wants children, trying 1 year ++
Social background:	Accountant, regular western diet
	Exercises 3 × week local gym
Medical background:	Frequent acute menstrual pain localised to the lower left quadrant.
	Pain persists despite taking OTC naproxen.
	Shy discussing sexual history.
	Occasional constipation, associated with pain in lower left quadrant.
	Trans-vaginal ultrasound showing 6cm cyst, likely of endometrial origin.
	Patient recovering post op from laparoscopic surgery (25/03/2018) – no complications.
Post op care:	Keep incisions clean and dry.
	Showering is permitted 26/03/2018
Mobility post op:	Patient can ambulate if confident.
	Driving is prohibited when on analgesics.
	Driving can be resumed 24-48 hrs after final dose analgesics.
	Sexual activity can be resumed 2 weeks post op.

Nursing management:	Encourage oral fluids.
	Patient may return to regular diet.
	Ambulation encouraged as per patient tolerance.
Medical progress:	Afebrile. Hct, Hgb, Plts, WBC, BUN, Cr, Na, K, Cl, HCO3, Glu all within normal limits. Patient sitting comfortably, alert, oriented × 4 (person, place, time, situation).
Assessment:	Good progress overall.
Discharge plan:	Patient to be discharged when can eat, ambulate, urinate independently.
	Patient must be discharged to someone who can drive them home.

Medical Writing Task 2

Using the information given to you in the case notes, write a letter of discharge to the patient's GP, Dr Stevens, Mill Street Surgery, Farnham, GU10 1HA.

In your answer:

- **Expand the relevant notes into complete sentences**
- **Do not use note form**
- **Use letter format**

The body of the letter should be approximately 180 – 200 words.

Nursing Writing Task 2

Using the information given to you in the case notes, write a letter summarising the patient's condition and communicating discharge instructions to the home health nurse, Joan Stevens, Millhouse Visiting Nurses Association, Farnham, GU10 1HA.

In your answer:

- **Expand the relevant notes into complete sentences**
- **Do not use note form**
- **Use letter format**

The body of the letter should be approximately 180 – 200 words.

Notes

You are a physician OR a nurse at a family medical practice. Ms Tabitha Taborlin is a 45-year-old patient at your practice.

Office: First Family Primary Care, 3959 Abalone Lane, Omaha

Patient Details

Name: Tabitha Taborlin (Ms)

Marital status: Single

Next of kin: Gregory Taborlin (69, father)

Date seen: 08 April, 2018

Diagnosis: Type 1 diabetes mellitus

Past medical history: Essential hypertension

Type 1 diabetes mellitus (non-compliant with insulin regimen)

Multiple episodes of diabetic ketoacidosis (DKA)

Social background: Schoolteacher, lives alone in apartment

Does not exercise, BMI 18.2 (underweight - 48kg)

Smokes moderately (2 cigs daily)

Medical background: Long history of Type 1 diabetes (since 7 y.o.) and noncompliance with insulin regimen.

On 45 units Lantus nightly and preprandial correctional scale Humalog with 12 unit nutritional baseline.

02/04/2018: admitted DKA (glucose 530 mmo/L)

IV fluids and insulin administered. Discharge stable - HbA1c.

Appointment today: Doing well since discharge.

Still not using insulin. Has insulin available.

Not following recommended diet.

Discussed diabetes education, necessity of glucose testing, insulin administration, smoking cessation education.

Discussed microvascular/macrovascular complications of diabetes.

Plan:	Discharge today – provide educational pamphlets and refills for Lantus and Humalog.
	Referral to endocrine specialist for stricter glycemic control and possible insulin pump.
	Follow-up in 1 month.

Medical Writing Task 3

Using the information given in the case notes, write a referral letter to Dr. Sharon Farquad, Endocrinologist at Endocrine Specialists and Associates, 115 Burke St. Omaha.

In your answer:

- **Expand the relevant notes into complete sentences**
- **Do not use note form**
- **Use letter format**

The body of the letter should be approximately 180 – 200 words.

Nursing Writing Task 3

Using the information given in the case notes, write a referral letter to the diabetic nurse educator, Dr. Hank Farquad, Certified Diabetes Educator at Endocrine Specialists and Associates, 115 Burke St. Omaha.

In your answer:

- **Expand the relevant notes into complete sentences**
- **Do not use note form**
- **Use letter format**

The body of the letter should be approximately 180 – 200 words.

Answers

1	Mr Walter Peters
2	Dr N Shah
3	the patient is being referred
4	New Canterbury Hospital, 1 Church Street, Canterbury
5	D N Shah Admitting Officer New Canterbury Hospital 1 Church Street Canterbury 15 September 2018 Dear Dr Shah

Writing Task 1

Medical Sample Response

Dr. Giovanni DiCoccio
Proudhurst Family Practice
231 Brightfield Avenue
Proudhurst

19/03/2018

Dear Dr. DiCoccio,

Re: Bethany Tailor (aged 35),

Your patient, Ms Tailor, admitted herself on 1 March 2018 with decompensated schizophrenia. She is now ready for discharge and follow-up at your clinic.

On admission, she was experiencing significant thought disorder, including thought blocking and latency. She was also exhibiting delusions and experiencing auditory command and visual hallucinations.

During her stay in hospital Ms Taylor was placed back on her medications, and her mental condition has stabilised and she is able to focus on her activities of daily living. Her insight is now good and judgment fair. Her nursing management in the hospital focused on compliance with her antipsychotic medications, behavioural control, and therapy. Since 10 March, she has not reported visual or auditory hallucinations.

Ms Tailor is on oral Risperidone 4mg nightly. Additional oral risperidone 1mg can be administered as needed twice daily for agitation or psychosis. She will be discharged from the hospital to her apartment where she lives alone. She will follow-up with you in order to continue her treatment of chronic schizophrenia and to avoid non-compliance of her medications or substance abuse.

If you have any queries, please contact me.

Yours sincerely,

Doctor

[183 words]

Nursing Sample Response

Maria DiCoccio
Proudhurst Mental Health Home
231 Brightfield Avenue
Proudhurst

19/03/2018

Dear Ms DiCoccio,

Re: Bethany Tailor (DOB: April 20, 2018),

Ms Bethany Tailor will be discharged to your facility today. She was admitted to the hospital on 1 March 2018 with decompensated schizophrenia, probably secondary to medication noncompliance and substance abuse.

On admission, she was experiencing significant thought disorder, including thought blocking and latency. She was also exhibiting delusions and experiencing auditory command and visual hallucinations.

After her stay in hospital and being placed back on her medications, her mental condition has stabilised and she is able to focus on her activities of daily living. She is demonstrating appropriate insight and judgement. Her nursing management in the hospital focused on compliance with her antipsychotic medications, behavioural control, and therapy. Since 10 March, she has not reported visual or auditory hallucinations.

Ms Tailor is on oral risperidone 4mg nightly. Additional oral risperidone 1mg can be administered as needed twice daily for agitation or psychosis. She is also prescribed levothyroxine 88 mcg by mouth for hypertension and hypothyroidism. She will require medication monitoring to avoid non-compliance of her medications or substance abuse.

If you have any queries, please contact me.

Yours sincerely,

Nurse

[191 words]

Writing Task 2

Medical Sample Response

Dr Stevens
Mill Street Surgery
Farnham
GU10 1HA

25 March 2018

Dear Dr Stevens,

Re: Mrs Sally Fletcher
         D.O.B 3/10/1993

Your patient, Sally Fletcher, was admitted to the surgical ward of Fairbanks Memorial Hospital on 25 March 2018 for the purpose of laparoscopic surgery to treat an endometrial cyst. She is now ready for discharge into the care of her husband.

When admitted, Sally had been suffering from painful periods over the past 3 years, which she had been attempting to treat with naproxen, but the pain persisted. An ultrasound scan revealed a cyst had formed in her abdomen. She arrived at the ward this morning and underwent laparoscopic surgery, which successfully located and removed a 6cm cyst from her abdomen without complication.

She has been advised to keep the incision sites clean and dry. She has received narcotic pain medication and has been advised that she is unable to drive while taking this medication. You should monitor her progress, and advise when to cease taking this medication. She may resume driving 24-48 hours after the last dose is taken.

Sally may resume her normal diet today, and is encouraged to drink plenty of fluids. She is also encouraged to walk as much as she can tolerate. Sexual activity can resume in two weeks.

If you have any questions please feel free to contact me.

Yours sincerely,

Doctor

[194 words]

Nursing Sample Response

Joan Stevens
Millhouse Visiting Nurses Association
Farnham
GU10 1HA

25 March 2018

Dear Ms Stevens,

Re: Mrs Sally Fletcher
        D.O.B 3/10/1993

Your patient, Sally Fletcher, was admitted to the surgical centre of Fairbanks Memorial Hospital on 25 March 2018 for laparoscopic surgery to treat an endometrial cyst. She is now ready for discharge.

When admitted, Sally had been suffering from painful periods over the past 3 years, caused by endometrial tissue present outside the uterus, which formed a cyst in her abdomen. She arrived at the centre this morning and underwent laparoscopic surgery to remove the cyst. The surgery successfully located and removed a 6cm cyst from her abdomen without complication.

She has been advised to keep the incision sites clean and dry. She has received narcotic pain medication and has been advised that she is unable to drive while taking this medication. She may resume driving 24-48 hours after the last dose is taken. She should be monitored for constipation, urinary retention and pain control while taking the narcotic.

Sally may resume her normal diet today, and is encouraged to drink plenty of fluids. She is also encouraged to walk as much as she can tolerate. Sexual activity can resume in two weeks.

If you have any questions please feel free to contact me.

Yours sincerely,

Nurse

[196 words]

Writing Task 3

Medical Sample Response

Dr. Sharon Farquad
Endocrinologist
Endocrine Specialists and Associates
115 Burke St.
Omaha

08/04/2018

Dear Dr. Farquad

Re: Tabitha Taborlin (aged 45)

Thank you for seeing Ms Tablorin as a new patient at Endocrine Specialists and Associates. She is a 45 year old female with a past medical history of essential hypertension and uncontrolled Type 1 diabetes mellitus.

Ms Tablorin was seen at my clinic today as a follow-up from a hospital admission for diabetic ketoacidosis with a glucose measure of 530 mmol/L. She has had multiple prior hospitalisations for the same issue. She also has a long history of being noncompliant with her insulin medications, which are 45 units of Lantus nightly, and preprandial correction scale Humalog with 12 units of nutritional baseline. Her HbA1c is 11.0%.

She has been educated multiple times on diabetes risks and complications, regarding her insulin regimen, exercise, diet, and tobacco cessation. However, she has continued to ignore these recommendations and her condition has progressively worsened. It is my recommendation that she seek a higher level of care, thus I refer her to your practice. Ms Tablorin would likely benefit from a stricter insulin regimen and glycemic monitoring, as well as an insulin pump for reliability of medication administration.

If you have any queries, please contact me.

Yours sincerely,

Doctor

[183 words]

Nursing Sample Response

Dr. Hank Farquad
Certified Diabetes Educator
Endocrine Specialists and Associates
115 Burke St.
Omaha
08/04/2018

Dear Dr. Farquad

Re: Tabitha Taborlin (aged 45),

Thank you for seeing Tabitha Taborlin as a new patient at Endocrine Specialists and Associates. She is a 45 year old female with a past medical history of essential hypertension and uncontrolled Type 1 diabetes mellitus.

Ms Tablorin was seen at my clinic today as a follow-up from a hospital admission for diabetic ketoacidosis with a glucose measure of 530 mmol/L. She has had multiple prior hospitalisations for the same issue. She has a long history of being noncompliant with her insulin medications, which are 45 units of Lantus nightly, and preprandial correction scale Humalog with 12 units of nutritional baseline. Her HbA1c is 11.0%.

Education was provided on diabetes risks and complications, using her insulin regimen, exercise, diet, and tobacco cessation. To date, she has not complied with these recommendations and her condition has progressively worsened. It is recommended that she seek a higher level of care, thus I refer her to your practice. Ms Tablorin would likely benefit from a stricter insulin regimen and glycemic monitoring, as well as an insulin pump for reliability of medication administration. She will require support with these changes to care.

If you have any queries, please contact me.

Yours sincerely,

Nurse

[191 words]

PART FIVE

The Speaking Section

Speaking Introduction

Section Overview

The OET Speaking Test is a face-to-face examination, between an interlocutor and you. Your Speaking Test will be specific to your healthcare profession; in this book, we will cover medical and nursing topics. In the Speaking Test, you will complete two role-plays, where you take the role of the healthcare professional, and the interlocutor takes the role of the patient, the carer or family member of the patient.

Speaking Strategies

- Treat the role-play as if you were with a real patient. Allow time to establish a relationship with the patient and ask for relevant information.

- Remember that the assessor is testing your ability to communicate effectively with patients in English; they are not testing your medical knowledge.

- Pay attention to the type of information you need to communicate to the patient, and adjust the way you communicate this information for different situations. If the patient is being given bad news, for example, you should show empathy and kindness.

- Don't memorise long answers. Anything the assessor thinks has been memorised will not be assessed.

- Use varied vocabulary which matches the needs of the patient and the context of the role-play. You need to show you can communicate with the patient in a variety of ways.

- Speak loudly, clearly and confidently so the interlocutor can hear you.

- Pronounce words as clearly and correctly as possible.

- Vary your intonation - your voice should rise and fall as a native speaker's would.

- Read the role-play card carefully, so you do not misunderstand or miss out on any of the topic or bullet points.

- Make brief notes for each point on the card. Include ideas and examples, but not full sentences.

- Try not to be nervous. Take a deep breath, smile and make eye contact as you begin your speaking task. While eye contact is not assessed, it can help you to feel more confident.

- Underline key words and phrases on the card, to assist you with the role-play.

- Don't be afraid to ask the interlocutor to clarify anything on the role-play card which is unclear. This can include the meaning or pronunciation of vocabulary and the context of the role-play. Ensure that any questions are asked before the role-play begins.

The Speaking Task

Introduction

The Speaking Test will take approximately 20 minutes. You will complete 2 role-plays, and will talk to the interlocutor for 5 minutes during each role-play. You will have 2 to 3 minutes to prepare for your role-play, using your role-play card before each role-play begins.

We will outline criteria that will be used to assess your Speaking Test in this chapter. When completing speaking tasks, make sure to keep the criteria provided in mind, and try to demonstrate your abilities in each individual section. We will give examples for how these criteria could be addressed in the speaking exam, however, we do not advise students to try to memorise these examples, or attempt to reproduce them word for word on Test Day.

Strategies

Getting ready to speak

The first step in the Speaking Test is to familiarise yourself with the role-play card. You will only be given one role-play card at a time, and you will not be given the interlocutor's role-play card. Be aware that the interlocutor's card will include information that is not included in your role-play card, so the card you are given will not fully prepare you for everything the patient will say, though it should give you a good idea of the outline that the conversation will take.

Below are two role-play cards. One is a Medical role-play, and the other is a Nursing role-play. Select the most appropriate role-play card, and use it to work through the following strategies.

Medical Task

CANDIDATE CARD NO. 1	MEDICINE
SETTING	General Practice
DOCTOR	A 44-year-old has been referred to your clinic due to high cholesterol and hypertension. They are frustrated about attending today.
TASK	• Find out what the patient thinks the purpose of the visit is today. • Explain the implications of high blood pressure and cholesterol on current and future health (e.g. strokes, heart attacks, kidney damage, etc). • Discuss cholesterol lowering drugs and anti-hypertensives and explain their benefits. • Find out about the patient's lifestyle (e.g. smoking and drinking habits) and advise the patient on how to improve his/her health (e.g. reducing smoking and alcohol consumption, joining a support group or seeing a counsellor, increasing exercise, etc.).

Nursing Task

CANDIDATE CARD NO. 2	NURSING
SETTING	General Practice
NURSE	A 67-year-old patient who has had hypertension with no known cause for many years has come in for a follow-up appointment. His/her blood pressure is moderately elevated today and he/she appears anxious.
TASK	• Find out if the patient has had any issues complying with the medications or exercising/eating healthily. • Explain the importance of medications for blood pressure control. • Discuss lifestyle changes that the patient can make to reduce their blood pressure (e.g. take the medications as prescribed, increase exercise, and eat a healthier diet, etc.).

Who is the patient?

The first thing you should identify is the type of patient you are going to talk with. Role-play cards will inform you of the key details about the patient and the reason for their appointment. You may also be told about the patient's emotions. You should take all of these pieces of information into consideration, and plan your approach accordingly. For example, if a patient is nervous or worried about a procedure, you will need to offer them reassurance.

Exercise

Match the following 3 patient descriptions with the most appropriate approach.

1. An 83 year old needs an MRI scan, and seems confused.
2. A 56 year old has terminal cancer, and is extremely upset.
3. A 24 year old has a viral infection and is impatiently requesting treatment.

    A Listen to what they have to say and find out what the patient wants to know.

    B Explain carefully, perhaps multiple times, while checking for understanding throughout the explanation.

    C Briefly outline the options available and recommend the optimal course of action.

Look at the description of your patient in the role-play card on the previous page. Take 30 seconds to consider how to best complete the tasks in bullet points and make brief notes below. Think about the language required to check for understanding.

_____

_____

_____

_____

_____

What do you need to find out?

Next, look at the bullet pointed tasks. At least one of these tasks will ask you to find out information from the patient. Identify what it is that you need to find out from the patient, and think of ways to rephrase the task into a question that would be appropriate for conversational English. Take another 30 seconds to think about rephrasing the information in the first bullet point of your role-play card, to turn this into appropriate questions. Your initial question should be an open question (for example, 'how are you feeling?'), which should then be followed up with more closed questions (for example, 'how long have you been experiencing these symptoms?').

_____

_____

_____

_____

_____

What do you need to tell the patient?

You will be required to provide your patient with necessary information about their condition, tests and course of treatment, and should ensure that the patient understands the information. What you need to communicate to the patient will be outlined in the bullet points of the role-play card. You may simply need to explain a point to the patient, or you may need to find out relevant information first, before tailoring your response to the patient's individual case. If you have a lot of information to communicate with the patient, you should break the information down into sections, so that you can check the patient's understanding for each section of information before moving on to the next section.

Speaking in English

Once your planning time is up, you should have a good idea of the structure your conversation will take. When speaking, you need to cover the following four linguistic criteria, to make sure that you are showing the assessor your ability to interact effectively. You need to show that you can have meaningful conversations with others in English. You should communicate confidently, take control of the interaction, lead the topic of conversation, and effectively complete the speaking task, by addressing all of the points in the task card and responding appropriately to the patient. While it is not essential that you cover all of the information in the 5 minutes provided for each conversation, you should not waste time or talk about points not mentioned in the role-play card.

Intelligibility

To score well in this criterion, you need to communicate in a way that can be easily heard and understood. The assessor will pay attention to your pronunciation, the rhythm you use when you speak, the stress you put on individual words, your intonation and your pitch. Avoid memorising large chunks of speech before the test, as this will sound unnatural. Instead, speak at an appropriate speed and clearly, allow your voice to rise and fall. Practise pronouncing words in English so that they sound the same as when a native English speaker says them. To address the first bullet pointed task in the nursing role-play card, you could say:

> "**Tell me** if you have had **any issues** following the **diet** that we discussed at your **last appointment**."

The words shown in bold in the sentence above should be stressed as they are the words which carry the meaning in the sentence. Stress is a slight increase in volume, and a slight increase in the sound length.

Fluency

This criterion addresses the rate and flow of your speech. You need to speak at an appropriate speed and carefully, think about the sentence you are going to say before saying it rather than saying something that you later need to correct. You should avoid overusing filler noises where possible, such as

> "Ah" "umm" "err"

and focus on speaking smoothly, linking your speech together, and pausing appropriately, for example, you might pause to separate different points you are making. You could say, for example

> *"First, we need to address your diet (pause) then, we can look at more invasive treatments."*

You can also pause for emphasis, or before beginning a new task on the role-play card, giving yourself a moment to think about what you will say next.

Appropriateness

This criterion assesses the appropriateness of your language and tone. Remember that you are speaking to a patient, not a medical professional, so you should explain any terms that they might not understand. For example, you would rephrase 'hypertension' in the role-player card to 'high blood pressure'. Your language and tone should also remain professional and confident, and you should adjust your tone to match the emotion of the patient, and the topic being discussed.

Resources of grammar and expression

You need to show that you can use grammar correctly and speak in a variety of tenses and sentence structures.

You should use grammatical devices such as chunking to make your speech clearer, and easier to understand. If you are giving the patient a large amount of information, you might say something like

> *"I'm going to discuss the various options available to you. The first is…"*

You should show that you can communicate information in a variety of ways. You might rephrase something you have already said, to make sure that the information can be understood by the patient. Make sure that you are using the correct word order when speaking, and do not omit words from your speech.

You should use the correct tense when speaking, to make sure that the patient knows if you are talking about something that has already happened, or something that they will need to do.

Speaking with the Patient

As OET is a test for healthcare professionals, as well as having a good command of the English language, you also need to be able to communicate effectively and responsively with patients. There are five clinical communication criteria which you will be assessed on. You do not have to address all parts of each of the 5 criteria to score well in the Speaking Test.

Relationship building

1. <u>Initiate the interaction appropriately</u>

You should start with an appropriate greeting. From the beginning of your interview, you should make the patient feel welcome, and at ease. Begin by introducing yourself, then give your role, and explain or remind the patient why the appointment has been scheduled. The following gives an appropriate example of a greeting:

> *"Hello, I'm Dr Albert, is it Margaret French? I'm one of the rheumatologists attached to the hospital. Your family doctor has asked me to see you about the joint problems you've been having"*

2. <u>Demonstrate an attentive and respectful attitude</u>

As the interview progresses, you should make sure to show that you are paying attention to the patient's needs and concerns, and show that you are listening to what the patient is telling you. This will help you to create a collaborative environment between you and the patient, and allow the patient to feel at ease with you. To meet these criteria, you could ask for the patient's permission to discuss topics that could potentially cause them to feel uncomfortable, check that the patient is comfortable with what is being discussed if there are any signs that they may not be, and show sensitivity when discussing anything that the patient may find embarrassing or personal. The following is an example of how you might demonstrate respect for the patient:

> *"What I would like to do is spend a few minutes with you now discussing your symptoms? Is that okay? Please let me know if you are feeling uncomfortable at any time"*

3. <u>Demonstrate a non-judgemental approach</u>

When the patient shares information, you should accept this information without reproach or judgement. Do not devalue or criticise the patient when they share their thoughts or behaviours, as this will discourage them from continuing to share information with you. You need to maintain respectful communication, so you should acknowledge the patient's emotions wherever possible. The following gives an example of how you might respond to a patient who has voiced concerns:

> *"So what worries you most is that the abdominal pain might be caused by cancer. I can understand that you would want to get that checked out."*

4. <u>Show empathy</u>

You should show the patient that you understand why they feel a certain way, if they are emotional in your interview. You should also be prepared to change your approach if there is an emotional element to your interview; for instance, if you have to break bad news. You can show that you are meeting these criteria through your words, but you can also show empathy through the tone of your voice, and through non-verbal sounds of agreement, sympathy and encouragement. You could demonstrate your empathy for the patient, by saying something like:

> *"I can see that your husband's memory loss has been very difficult for you to cope with; I imagine I would feel similarly if the same thing happened to me".*

Understanding and incorporating the patient's perspective

In the Speaking Test, you need to show that you're putting the patient at the centre of the conversation, planning your speech around how you expect the patient to react and modifying your speech if they react in a different way. Follow the next three steps to make sure you are using the information your patient provides to alter your conversation.

1. <u>Elicit and explore the patient's concerns</u>

Encourage the patient to give their thoughts and opinions about their condition. Don't simply ask them to list their symptoms, but also explore what they think might be the cause. For example, you could say:

> *"Did you have any thoughts about what might be causing your symptoms?"*

or, to get an idea of what the patient might be feeling, you could say:

> *"Was there anything particular you were concerned about?"*

If the patient has not explained something fully, or you want to explore something further, you can do this by saying something like:

> *"You mentioned that you were concerned about the effect the illness might have on your work, could you tell me more about that?"*

2. Pick up on patient cues, and react accordingly

Alongside encouraging the patient to provide information, you will also need to show that you're taking this information into consideration, and shaping the conversation around what the patient is telling you. Many test-takers do not score well in the Speaking Test because they try to follow a specific structure for the conversation, which they do not adapt and alter according to new information provided by the patient. Do not memorise long dialogue to use on Test Day. Instead, practise reacting to new information, and incorporating it into your speech. When reacting to emotional patients, you might say something like:

> *"You used the word worried, could you tell me more about what you are worried about?"*

or, when patients show emotion, but do not tell you that they feel a certain way, you could say, for example:

> *"I sense that you are not happy with the explanations you've been given in the past."*

3. Relate your explanations to the ideas, concerns and expectations you have elicited from the patient

To show the patient that you are using the information they've given you to structure and guide your speech, you should let the patient know that their words have been heard. If a patient gives new information that changes the structure of your conversation, you could indicate this by saying something like:

> *"As you say you're having trouble sleeping at the moment, let's talk about things that might help you address this before we move on."*

If, on the other hand, the patient provides information that does not alter the conversation, you can still acknowledge their input by saying something like:

> *"You mentioned earlier that you were concerned that you had angina. Angina is a very particular kind of pain, which relates to several underlying conditions. Is it alright if I ask you a few more questions to rule out muscular pain?"*

Providing Structure

1. Sequence the interview purposefully and logically

You should structure the interview clearly and efficiently. Begin by greeting the patient, discuss why they're seeing you today, then tackle each bullet point, one by one. After you have provided an explanation, or completed a series of questions, check that the patient has no further questions and has understood you before moving on. While making notes on your role-play card in the preparation time, look through what you have to talk about, and think about how you might connect the bullet points to one another in your speech, so that your speaking flows logically – this relates to signposting.

2. Signpost changes in topic

Signposts function as a pause between topics and allow you to check for understanding and ask for permission to discuss topics. They also allow you to summarise information given by the interlocutor (this relates to later criteria). When moving from one topic to the next, you need to make it clear to the patient what you will discuss. After greeting the patient, you should outline the topic that will be discussed before getting into details. Whenever you move onto a different topic, tell the patient what you are moving on to talk about next. You might start to discuss a topic by saying something like this:

> "Since we haven't met before, it will help me to learn something about your past medical history. Can we do that now?"

After a patient has finished telling you about something, you might outline what you want to discuss next by saying something like this:

> "You mentioned two areas there that are obviously important, first the joint problems and the tiredness, and second, how you are going to cope with your kids. Could I start by just asking a few more questions about the joint pains, and then we can come back to your difficulties with the children?"

Signposting any changes in topic helps the patient to keep track of what's being discussed and gives a clearer structure to your discussion.

3. Use organising techniques in your explanations

There are a number of different ways that you might organise your explanations. Again, your primary concern when organising your explanations should be to make your speech as clear and digestible to the patient as possible. To help the patient understand, and to make it easier for them to remember information discussed at a later date, it can be helpful to divide what you will talk about into categories, and inform the patient of these categories before you go into more detail about each point. For example, you could say:

> "There are three important things I want to explain. Firstly I want to tell you what I think is wrong, secondly, what tests we should do, and thirdly, what the treatment may be."

The use of categorisation above helps to structure the discussion you will have, so that the patient can understand what will happen next. When you go into more detail, you should use a technique called chunking. This is when you deliver information in chunks, leaving clear gaps between each piece of information, before moving on to the next one. You may also find it helpful to use a technique called labelling. Labelling allows you to highlight significant information to the patient. For example, you could say:

> "It is particularly important that you remember this…"

Once you have explained all of the points you wanted to cover, it can also be useful to repeat and summarise the most important points to the patient. You could say, for example:

> "So just to recap: we have decided to treat this as a fungal infection with a cream that you put on twice a day for two weeks and if it is not better by then, you are going to come back to see me."

Repeating and summarising information makes it easier for the patient to store the information in their memory, and improves their ability to recall this information later. After you have summarised the information, you can check for the patient's understanding, which meets other criteria discussed later.

Exercise

Spend one minute thinking about the structure of the conversation that will take place, covered in the role-play card above. Think about how you will guide the conversation, and how you might rephrase the tasks into conversational English.

_____

_____

_____

_____

_____

Information Gathering

It's important to get as much relevant information from the patient as you can. If you've followed the steps outlined above, you should have created an environment where your patient feels comfortable sharing information with you. Now, you should read through the next 5 points to make sure you're listening actively to the patient, and gathering necessary and relevant information. This criterion asses your ability to address the way the patient is thinking and feeling, rather than your medical accuracy.

1. Facilitate the patient's narrative

When the patient is talking, you need to show that you are paying attention to them and following their speech, without interrupting them, or halting the flow of their narrative.

You can demonstrate that you are listening by using a number of techniques:

- When the patient pauses during their speech, don't try to start talking immediately, and don't interrupt the patient if they're still talking. Instead, wait until the patient has finished, and pause to consider what they have said before responding.

- You can use short verbal and non-verbal sounds of encouragement while the patient is speaking to show that you are paying attention. Examples include:

  "Um", "uh-huh", "I see"

- As the patient reveals information, you should show that you're taking this on board by echoing the patient, or repeating key phrases and words from their speech, such as

  "chest pain?"

or

  "not coping?"

Similarly, to show a greater understanding of what the patient is saying, you can rephrase what the patient is saying into your own words, or suggest an interpretation for what the patient is communicating. You could say, for example:

  "Are you thinking that when John gets even more ill, you won't be strong enough to nurse him at home by yourself?"

2. <u>Use open questions at the beginning and closed questions as the interview progresses</u>

At the beginning of your interview, you should ask the patient open questions, to find out as much general information as possible. The following are examples of open questions:

"Start at the beginning and take me through what has been happening…"

"How have you been feeling since your operation…?"

"Tell me about your headaches."

As the conversation develops and you have a better idea of the information you need from the patient, your questions can become more directed, but should remain open. At this stage, you could ask:

"What makes your headaches better or worse?"

Once the patient has provided enough general information about their condition, you can move to more specific, closed questions to get further information.

"Do you ever wake up with this headache in the morning?"

3. <u>Avoid compound questions and leading questions</u>

To ensure that you are receiving reliable information, you should avoid influencing your patient when you ask questions, or asking multiple questions at once. An example of a compound question is:

"Have you ever had chest pain or felt short of breath?"

The patient may simply respond 'yes' or 'no', even if the answer does not relate to both their experience of chest pain and their experience of shortness of breath. You should always break compound questions up and ask one question at a time.

Leading questions include assumptions. This makes it more difficult for the patient to contradict the assumption. Avoid asking leading questions in your interview, such as:

"You've lost weight, haven't you? or "you haven't had any ankle swelling?"

These questions are unlikely to provide you with reliable information.

4. <u>Clarify statements that are vague or require amplification</u>

If patients respond to your questions without providing enough information, or with a response that could be interpreted in a number of different ways, it is important to ask the patient to explain what they mean. You might ask, for example:

"Could you explain what you mean by light-headed?"

If the patient says something that requires further amplification, for instance, if they appear to describe a symptom, but you'd like to get a clearer idea of what they are actually experiencing, you can look for amplification by asking something like:

"When you say dizzy, do you mean that the room seems to actually spin round?"

Don't move on to discuss something else until you're comfortable that you've understood what the patient has said. Remember that patients may be less precise with their vocabulary, so it is important to clarify their statements.

5. Summarise information to encourage the patient to correct or give more information

Once the patient has finished discussing a topic, and you think that you have all of the relevant information you need, you should give a brief overview of what the patient has told you, and ask the patient to confirm this, and provide more information. You might say, for example:

> *"Can I just see if I've got this right – you've had indigestion before, but for the last few weeks you've had increasing problems with a sharp pain at the front of your chest. This has been accompanied by wind and acid and it's stopping you from sleeping. It's made worse by drink and you were wondering if the painkillers were to blame. Is that right?"*

Once you've summarised the information, and if the patient has agreed, pause for a moment longer, to allow the patient to provide any additional information, or to correct or alter part of the information.

Information Giving

After the patient has finished providing information, and you have gathered everything you need, and confirmed that it is correct, it is your turn to provide information to the patient. Read through the next 5 points, to make sure that you explain information as effectively as possible. Remember, it is not about giving the most medically accurate explanations possible, but it is about checking that the patient has understood the information.

1. Establish what the patient already knows

The first step in explaining information is to understand what the patient is aware of already, so that you can focus on explaining things they don't know, and avoid going over things they're already familiar with. Don't assume that the patient is familiar with their illness or treatment, as they may not be. To establish how much the patient knows, you might ask something like:

> *"It would be helpful for me to understand a little of what you already know about diabetes so that I can try to fill in any gaps for you."*

> *"Based on your blood test results, we need to discuss ways to lower your cholesterol. What do you know about Lipitor?"*

2. Pause periodically when giving information, using the patient's response to guide next steps

Once you are aware of what the patient needs to know, you can begin to explain information to them. Make sure you take breaks throughout your explanation, allowing the patient time to ask questions before moving on. For example, you might say something like

> *"So really, given the symptoms you have described and the very typical way that you wheeze more after exercise and at night, I feel reasonably confident that what you are describing is asthma and that we should consider ways we might treat it. (Pause) How does that sound so far?"*

3. <u>Encourage patients to contribute reactions and feelings</u>

You should make sure that the patient feels comfortable with what you are explaining so that you can address this before moving on. Patients who are feeling uncomfortable, confused or distressed may find it more difficult to take in information, so you should check their reactions to the information from time to time. You could do this by asking something like:

> *"What questions does that leave you with, have you any concerns about what I have said?"*

4. <u>Check that the patient has understood</u>

As well as checking the patient's emotional reactions to the information, you also need to make sure that the patient understands what you are explaining to them. You can evaluate the patient's understanding by asking them to repeat the information that you have just given them. For example:

> *"I know I've given you a lot of information today and I'm concerned that I might not have made it very clear – it would help me if you repeated back to me what we have discussed so far so I can make sure we are on the same track."*

Make sure that the patient covers everything that you have explained, and if any information is missed in the patient's recap, remind them of the information, and check that they understand this information before moving on.

5. <u>Discover what further information the patient needs</u>

After confirming that the patient has understood everything that you have explained, you should find out if there is anything else that the patient wants to know. You could ask, for example:

> *"Are there any other questions you'd like me to answer or any points I haven't covered?"*

Exercise

Ask a friend or family member to use the role-play card on the following pages (they should make sure they choose the role-play card that corresponds with your role-play card earlier in the chapter, either medical or nursing) and play the role of the patient, while you play the role of the healthcare professional. Record the audio (you can use your mobile phone or laptop to do this) so that you can review it later, and set a timer for 5 minutes.

Nursing Task

ROLEPLAYER CARD NO. 1	NURSING
SETTING	General Practice
PATIENT	You are a 67-year-old and have had high blood pressure for many years. Your blood pressure was well controlled with medication and diet/exercise when you were working, but since retiring 2 years ago you have let your routine lapse. You are nervous about seeing the nurse because you don't want to be judged for not managing your blood pressure correctly.
TASK	• When asked, reluctantly admit that you haven't been taking your medication, exercising, and eating healthily all the time. Explain that you have been feeling fine and don't think that your blood pressure is an issue.

• Ask the nurse why you have to take so many medications.

• Be resistant to making any changes to your lifestyle initially, but eventually agree to the nurse's suggestions. |

Medicine Task

ROLEPLAYER CARD NO. 2	MEDICINE
SETTING	General Practice
PATIENT	You are a 44-year-old who has recently been told that both your cholesterol and blood pressure are high. You don't really want to take any medication. You don't really want to change your lifestyle because your health has been fine.
TASK	• Tell the doctor that the nurse referred you but you think you're wasting everybody's time because your health is fine.
	• Be dismissive of the doctor's warning about the future. Your friend has high blood pressure and cholesterol and they are fine.
	• If asked, tell the doctor that you are reluctant to take statins because you have heard that they can cause problems with your joints.
	• If the doctor asks, divulge your alcohol and smoking history (10 cigarettes per day for the past 25 years, 2 pints of beer each night). Reluctantly agree to reduce how much you drink and smoke.

Once you've completed the speaking exercise, look through the assessment criteria again, and evaluate whether or not you met each criteria. Think about how you could have improved your speaking, and make notes on your weakest areas. Practise the skills necessary to meet the criteria, then try completing the speaking role-plays at the end of this chapter. You should always record yourself, and listen back over your speaking after you've completed the role-plays.

With each new speaking task, you should improve your speaking abilities further, until your speaking level is sufficiently improved for you to apply to the test situation on Test Day.

Speaking Practice Set

Use the 4 speaking role-plays on the following pages to practise your speaking skills with a friend, relative or colleague. Give yourself 2 to 3 minutes to prepare for the role-plays, using only your candidate role-play card, then record yourself speaking for 5 minutes. Once you have finished each role-play, assess your abilities using the speaking criteria in this chapter. When practising, you should only read the candidate card, as you will not see the roleplayer card in the test. You might find it helpful to photocopy and print these task cards onto one page, and then fold it in half, so you can focus on the candidate card while you're getting ready to speak.

Medical Task Cards

CANDIDATE CARD NO. 3	MEDICINE

SETTING	Pain Medicine Clinic
DOCTOR	This 32-year-old patient has been attending your pain medicine clinic for several years and has been prescribed opioids (painkillers) due to a workplace injury. He/she is requesting an early refill, but your clinic has a no early refill policy.
TASK	• Find out why the patient is requesting an early refill.
	• Discuss the clinic's no early-refill policy and the reason behind it (abuse of opioid medication).
	• Tactfully explain that you cannot write a refill, but that you can help the patient manage their pain in other ways (e.g. topical creams, over-the-counter pain killers, anti-depressants like Cymbalta, etc.).
	• Try and reassure the patient. Explain that if the pain becomes unbearable, they should visit the Emergency Department.

ROLE-PLAYER CARD NO. 3	MEDICINE

SETTING	Pain Medicine Clinic
PATIENT	You are 32 and have been attending a pain medicine clinic for several years due to a workplace injury. You are on short-acting and long-acting painkillers, which are refilled every month. However, this weekend, someone stole your medications. You now have none and your refill is two weeks away. You are hoping to get an early refill but are nervous that the clinic has a policy of not replacing stolen medication.
TASK	• Explain your situation to the doctor and express your anxiety about having to be in pain again.
	• Explain that you understand the provider's policy and the rationale behind it, but are asking for leniency given the first-time nature of this incident.
	• Insist that you should be able to obtain a refill.
	• Become anxious about managing your pain. Be difficult to reassure.

CANDIDATE CARD NO. 4	MEDICINE

SETTING	General Hospital Emergency Department
DOCTOR	You are talking to a 54-year old patient, who has been recently diagnosed with adenocarcinoma (lung cancer). A chest X-ray was completed in the Emergency Department and reveals bilateral opacifications (an underlying condition such as pneumonia, oedema, haemorrhage, etc. is blocking air getting into the lungs). You are concerned that the patient may be suffering from a malignant pleural effusion (fluid in the lungs) and require a thoracentesis (removal of the fluid via a needle).
TASK	• Find out about the patient's concerns regarding their diagnosis.
	• Share with the patient the X-ray findings and the possible reasons behind his/her shortness of breath.
	• Reassure the patient regarding the likely course of treatment: ultrasound to see if he/she has a pleural effusion with chemotherapy to be organised when the other symptoms resolve.
	• Find out what further information the patient needs. Refer the patient to a counsellor and explain the possible treatment options (diuretics, thoracentesis, no treatment, etc).

ROLEPLAYER CARD NO. 4	MEDICINE
SETTING	General Hospital Emergency Department
PATIENT	You are a 54-year-old patient who has been recently diagnosed with lung cancer. You visited the Emergency Department (ED) and explained to the doctors that you can't catch your breath and taking deep breaths causes chest tightness. You are scared and worried because you went through cancer recovery before and had chemotherapy and radiation to treat an aggressive B-cell lymphoma. You are worried that you may not tolerate more chemotherapy and this new shortness of breath is related to your lung cancer.
TASK	• Express concern regarding chemotherapy and your new symptoms. • Ask if your shortness of breath may be caused by your lung cancer. • Ask if chemotherapy is necessary and what you can expect if you have chemotherapy treatment. • When asked, explain that you don't really want more procedures; you just want to go home. You would like to speak to a counsellor. Reluctantly listen to the doctor's options.

Nursing Task Cards

ROLEPLAYER CARD NO. 5	NURSING

SETTING	Outpatient Mental Health Clinic
NURSE	This 24-year-old patient was recently prescribed lithium for his/her bipolar disorder but is now worried about continuing with this drug. He/she is would like to know more about the medication, including its indications, side effects, and monitoring.
TASK	• Find out the why the patient is concerned and if they are experiencing side effects. • Explain how lithium works (e.g. very effective mood stabiliser) and that they will have to take it forever, although the dose may be adjusted. • Go over some side effects with the patient while providing reassurance (e.g. acne and hair loss are common but other side effects like seizures are rare). • Check that the patient has understood your explanations and find out what further advice they need. Provide further reassurance that they are doing the right thing.

ROLEPLAYER CARD NO. 5	NURSING

SETTING   Outpatient Mental Health Clinic

PATIENT   You are 24 years old and have a diagnosis of bipolar mood disorder. The psychiatrist has prescribed you lithium as a mood stabiliser. You have been taking it for a week and done some research online. You are worried now because everyone appears to report having negative side effects on the medication. You would like to know if you should continue to take the medication, how it works and what side effects to watch out for.

TASK
- Explain your worry over what you have read online and your concern about the safety of continuing this medicine.

- Ask how it treats your condition. Will you need to take it forever?

- Find out what sort of side effects are typical. How likely is it they will occur?

- Be reluctant to continue taking lithium. Eventually agree to the nurse's advice.

CANDIDATE CARD NO. 6	NURSING

SETTING	Rehab Facility
PATIENT	You have been asked by a family member to speak to a patient who is recovering from a subarachnoid haemorrhage (SAH) (bleeding between the skull and the cortex). The patient is concerned that a full recovery will not occur and that another SAH is inevitable.
TASK	• Find out the specifics of the patient's concerns. Reassure the patient that fatigue will lessen and physical endurance and memory will improve as the brain continues to heal. • Explain that some patients are able to go back to work/live independently. • Discuss how the patient could live independently: e.g., assistive devices (walker or cane, grab bars in bathroom), visual cues to trigger memory (post-it notes, pictures), setting alarm clocks to serve as reminders (time for medications, phone calls, etc.). • Stress the importance of taking BP (blood pressure) medications as prescribed. Suggest that the patient use a 7-day pill organiser.

ROLE-PLAYER CARD NO. 6	NURSING

SETTING	Rehab Facility
PATIENT	You are 49-years-old and recovering from a subarachnoid haemorrhage (SAH) (bleeding between the skull and the cortex) that occurred three months ago. You were discharged from an acute care facility to a rehab facility yesterday. You were told that you will continue to improve over the next 12 months, but you are concerned about the highest level of functioning that you will achieve. You also would like to know how to prevent another SAH.
TASK	• Tell the nurse that you are concerned that you will not regain your stamina, financial control or be able to live independently. • Ask the nurse if patients are ever able to live independently and go back to work after recovering from a SAH. • Ask the nurse how you can maintain good BP (blood pressure) to prevent another SAH.

Answers

1	B
2	A
3	C

PART SIX

The Practice Test

Listening Section

 Play **Track 21** to complete the Listening Test.

Listening Test

This test has three parts. In each part you'll hear a number of different extracts.

You'll hear each extract **ONCE ONLY**.

At the end of the test you'll have five minutes to transfer your answers onto the separate answer sheet.

Part A

In this part of the test, you'll hear two different extracts. In each extract, a health professional is talking to a patient.

For **questions 1 to 24**, complete the notes with information you hear in the recording.

Extract 1: Questions 1 to 12

You hear a foundation doctor talking to a recently admitted patient called Roy Miller. For **questions 1 to 12**, complete the notes with a word or short phrase.

Name	Roy Miller

Reasons for admission	• shortness of breath
	   – difficulty walking **(1)**_____, often becomes short of breath
	   – breathlessness has increased
	• coughing and wheezing
	   – sounds like '**(2)**_____' and hasn't improved
	   – worse when **(3)**_____, preventing sleep
	   – coughing up phlegm, described as **(4)**_____ in colour
	   – phlegm has gradually darkened over the week
	• suffering hot and cold spells, feels **(5)**_____

Medical history	• diagnosed with **(6)**_____ last year • was a **(7)**_____, stopped six years ago • occasionally suffers from gout (treated with **(8)**_____) • arthritis located in **(9)**_____
Medication	• using **(10)**_____ more frequently • takes a statin for **(11)**_____ • occasionally uses paracetamol for arthritis • **(12)**_____ causes an allergic reaction

Extract 2: Questions 13 to 24

You hear an optometrist talking to a patient called Marsha Samarina. For **questions 13 to 24**, complete the notes with a word or short phrase.

Patient	Marsha Samarina
Description of initial symptoms	• pain in eye, felt like something was **(13)**_____ • noticed headache • eye was '**(14)**_____' profusely (compares to chopping onions) • roommate noticed that eye was **(15)**_____, took to ER • pain was severe, unable to **(16)**_____
Initial GP treatment	• unable to identify cause, performed **(17)**_____ test • GP suggested possibility of **(18)**_____
Optometrist treatment	• given **(19)**_____ for pain-relief • eye exam showed **(20)**_____

At home treatment	• advised to avoid wearing contacts
	• prescribed:
	  – **(21)**_____ - using twice daily
	  – and **(22)**_____ less often, finds application unpleasant
	• also taking **(23)**_____ for pain relief

Current condition	• condition has improved • pain caused by **(24)**_____

Part B

In this part of the test, you'll hear six different extracts. In each extract, you'll hear people talking in a different healthcare setting.

For **questions 25 to 30**, choose the answer (**A**, **B** or **C**) which fits best according to what you hear.

25. You hear two doctors discuss the transfer of care for a patient.

    The patient's CURB-65 score means that he will

    (A) be transferred from the Emergency Department.

    (B) receive additional medication and treatment.

    (C) be treated as an out-patient.

26. You hear a speech pathologist talking to the wife of a patient who has recently suffered a stroke.

    What does she want to know about her husband's condition?

    A how long it will take him to make a full recovery

    B whether his communication issues will improve

    C what she can do to speed the healing process

27. You hear a trainee doctor asking a senior colleague about chest tubes.

    What is the senior colleague doing?

    A explaining how to use them correctly

    B recommending an alternative to them

    C demonstrating what can go wrong with them

28. You hear a pharmacist talking to a customer about pain relief.

    What has the customer been misinformed about?

    A the stock of medication in the pharmacy

    B the usefulness of a type of pain relief

    C the availability of a medicine

29. You hear a trainee nurse receiving feedback from his tutor

    What does she explain?

    A listening to a patient's concerns is essential

    B how to become more self-assured when interacting with patients

    C the importance of providing adequate emotional support to patients

30. You hear two doctors planning their patient-care schedule

    What is their priority?

    A identifying the patients at greatest risk

    B dealing with patients who need tests arranging

    C ensuring that all patients have key documentation

Part C

In this part of the test, you'll hear two different extracts. In each extract, you'll hear health professionals talking about aspects of their work.

For **questions 31 to 42**, choose the answer (**A**, **B** or **C**) which fits best according to what you hear.

Extract 1: Questions 31 to 36

You hear an interview with Dr Matthew Leach, who's talking about meningitis caused by *Neisseria meningitides*.

31. Dr Leach says that during the onset of meningitis, many patients

    (A) do not realise they are unwell.

    (B) mistake the illness for something else.

    (C) experience life-threatening symptoms.

32. Dr Leach says that meningitis is common in college students because of their

    (A) poor hygiene habits.

    (B) proximity to new people.

    (C) weakened immune systems.

33. Why does Dr Leach say the patient didn't seek treatment sooner?

    (A) He was unsure of what to do.

    (B) He didn't think he needed treatment.

    (C) He was trying to finish his assignments.

34. Dr Leach began treating for meningitis before receiving the spinal fluid results because

    (A) the illness progresses rapidly.

    (B) the treatment is the same for all causes.

    (C) the test results did not affect the diagnosis.

35. Dr Leach explains that meningitis is more likely to cause long term after-effects if

    (A) it is not accurately diagnosed.

    (B) patients do not seek treatment quickly.

    (C) reactions to the virus are extremely severe.

36. Dr Leach advises those who think they may be infected with meningitis to

    (A) get vaccinated at the earliest opportunity.

    (B) avoid people who may be suffering from the virus.

    (C) take precautions to prevent others from becoming ill.

Extract 2: Questions 37 to 42

You hear a presentation given by a clinical psychiatrist called Dr Evalina Houghton about agitated patients in an emergency setting.

37. Dr Houghton says that patients in the ED are more likely to be agitated as they are likely to

    A suffer from untreated health problems.

    B have been given bad news recently.

    C require medical help frequently.

38. Dr Houghton explains that creating space between the patient and the provider

    A enables both parties to remain calm.

    B encourages the patient to exit the room.

    C reduces the likelihood of the provider being injured.

39. Why does Dr Houghton encourage providers to speak slowly?

    A to ensure the patient understands what is being said

    B to give other members of staff time to prepare

    C to give the patient an opportunity to speak

40. What approach does Dr Houghton suggest for patients suffering from delusions?

    A agree with the patient completely

    B acknowledge the patient's emotions

    C explain why their delusions are false

41. Dr Houghton suggests that choices given to the patient should

    A avoid upsetting the patient by remaining positive.

    B maintain the patient's trust by being realisable.

    C be limited in order to prevent confusion.

42. Dr Houghton recommends that when the patient is calm they should

    A be removed from the ED ward.

    B understand why their behaviour was inappropriate.

    C be encouraged to explain what caused their reaction.

END OF LISTENING

Reading Section

Part A

TIME: 15 minutes
- Look at the four texts, **A – D**, in the Text Booklet.
- For each question, **1 – 20**, look through the texts, **A – D**, to find the relevant information.
- Write your answers in the spaces provided in this **Question Paper**.
- Answer all the questions within the 15-minute time limit.

Asthma: Questions

Questions 1 – 6

For each question below, **1 – 6**, decide which text (**A**, **B**, **C** or **D**) the information comes from.

You may use any letter more than once.

In which text can you find information about

1. relaxation techniques for those suffering from an asthma attack? _____

2. measuring the respiration abilities in patients with asthma? _____

3. identifying the intensity of asthma attacks in patients? _____

4. the procedure to follow when treating an asthma attack? _____

5. symptoms of asthma in patients? _____

6. how to diagnose asthma in patients? _____

Questions 7 – 12

Complete each of the sentences, **7 – 12**, with a word or short phrase from one of the texts. Each answer may include words, numbers or both. Your answers should be correctly spelled.

7. To understand how severe an asthma attack is, **(7)**_____ must be measured, in addition to PEF.

8. For patients who do not respond to therapy, an IV of **(8)**_____ can be used to treat severe asthma attacks.

9. Nitric oxide testing can be used to determine **(9)**_____ in patients.

10. A patient suffering from arrhythmia and a peak expiratory flow of greater than 33% would be diagnosed with **(10)**_____ asthma attacks.

11. Spirometry tests that contain **(11)**_____ typically last for half an hour.

12. **(12)**_____ can cause neutrophilic inflammation in patients with asthma.

Questions 13 – 20

Answer each of the questions, **13 – 20**, with a word or short phrase from one of the texts. Each answer may include words, numbers or both. Your answers should be correctly spelled.

13. How often should patients be advised to practice breathing exercises?

_____

14. How often should patients with a peak expiratory flow of less than 75% be given 10 mg of salbutamol?

_____

15. When should patients be given 2mg of magnesium sulfate?

_____

16. Which patients will typically need to run when completing spirometry tests?

_____

17. What should staff do when assessing a patient suffering from a life-threatening panic attack?

_____

18. Which lung function test is helpful for understanding how the patient responds to treatment?

_____

19. What sort of noise might patients with asthma make when breathing?

_____

20. What is used to measure peak expiratory flow rate?

_____

Asthma: Texts

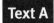

Establishing the severity of an acute asthma attack

	Moderate asthma	Severe asthma	Life-threatening asthma	
	Measure PEF and arterial saturation			
	PEF >50-75% predicted	PEF 33-50% predicted	PEF <33% predicted	
Adults	• SpO$_2$ ≥92% • PEF > 50-75% predicted • No features of acute severe asthma	• SpO$_2$ ≥92% • PEF < 50% predicted • RR ≥ 25/min • HR ≥ 110/min • difficulty talking	• SpO$_2$ ≥92% • silent chest • cyanosis • poor respiratory effort	• arrhythmia • hypotension • exhaustion • altered consciousness

Asthma sufferers of any severity may also experience the following:

- shortness of breath
- coughing

- tightness or pain in the chest
- a whistling sound when exhaling

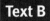

Lung Function Tests in Asthma

Asthma tests should be undertaken to diagnose and aid management of the condition. This is particularly important in asthma, because it presents slightly differently with each patient. Spirometry is the most important test, however several different types of test are available:

- **Peak expiratory flow rate (PEFR):** this is the maximum flow rate during exhalation, after full lung inflation. Diurnal variation in PEFR is a good measure of asthma and useful to the long-term management of patients and the response to treatment. Monitor PEFR over 2-4 weeks in adults if there is uncertainty about diagnosis. It is measured with a peak flow meter - a small, handheld device - into which the patient blows, giving a reading in l/min.

- **Spirometry:** measures volume and flow of air that can be exhaled or inhaled during normal breathing. Asthma can be diagnosed with a >15% improvement in FEV1 or PEFT following bronchodilator inhalation. Alternatively, consider FEV1/FVC < 70% as a positive result for obstructive airway disease. A spirometry test usually takes less than 10 minutes, but will last about 30 minutes if it includes reversibility testing.

  - **Direct bronchial challenge test with histamine or methacholine:** in this test, patients breathe in a bronchoconstrictor. The degree of narrowing can be quantified by spirometry. Asthmatics will react to lower doses, due to existing airway hyperactivity.

  - **Exercise tests:** these are often used for the diagnosis of asthma in children. The child should run 6 minutes (on a treadmill or other) at a workload sufficient to increase their heart rate > 160/min. Spirometry is used before and after the exercise - an FEV1 decrease > 10% indicates exercise-induced asthma.

- **Allergy testing:** can be useful if year-round allergies trigger a patient's asthma. This will be recommended if inhaled corticosteroids are not controlling symptoms. Three different tests are used to measure the patient's reaction to allergens: nitric oxide testing, sputum eosinophils and blood eosinophils.

Text C

Patients with asthma of any severity may find their attacks panic-inducing. Remember that the patient's struggle to breathe can cause stress, panic and a feeling of helplessness. There is a strong link between people who suffer from asthma and those who experience panic attacks. Staff must keep this in mind when treating patients with asthma, as some sufferers will require additional emotional support.

Patients may find breathing exercises beneficial. Advise patients to practice daily, to allow these exercises to become habitual. When experiencing an attack, patients should make a conscious effort to relax their muscles and maintain steady breathing. Advise patients to breathe deeply in through the nose and out through the mouth.

Smokers are at a higher risk of developing both panic attacks and asthma. In addition, smoking can irritate the airways in patients with asthma, causing neutrophilic inflammation, and exacerbating breathing problems in those with asthma. Ensure that patients who smoke are fully aware of the risks of smoking with asthma.

Text D

Management of Acute Asthma

Rapid treatment and reassessment is of paramount importance. It is sometimes difficult to assess severity. Maintaining a calm atmosphere is helpful to resolving an acute asthmatic attack.

Assess the severity of the attack

1. Check peak expiratory flow (PEF)
2. Is the patient able to speak?
3. Check respiratory rate (RR)
4. Check pulse rate
5. Check O_2 saturation
   If life-threatening or severe: warn ICU

Immediate Treatment

1. Maintain O_2 saturation with oxygen (94-98%)
2. Salbutamol 5mg with O_2 (nebulised)
3. Ipratropium 5mg every 6 hours if severe
4. Prednisolone 40-50mg PO or Hydrocortisone 100mg IV

Every 15 minutes: re-assess

1. PEF < 75%: salbutamol repeated every 15-30 minutes, or 10mg every hour continuously.
   If not yet given, add ipratropium.
2. Monitor ECG and check for arrhythmias
3. Magnesium Sulfate ($MgSO_4$), 1.2-2g IV over 20 minutes is an option in severe cases not responding to therapy

No improvement

1. Refer to ICU for ventilator support
2. Escalation of medical therapy
3. Check for:
   – PEF deteriorating
   – hypoxia
   – hypercapnia
   – ABG: low pH or high H^+
   – Exhaustion
   – Drowsiness and confusion
   – Respiratory arrest

Improvement within 15 – 30 minutes

1. Continue salbutamol every 4-6 hours
2. Check peak PEF and O_2 saturation
3. Prednisolone 40-50 mg PO OD for 5-7 days
4. If PEF>75% an hour after treatment, consider discharge with follow-up

Part B

In this part of the test, there are six short extracts relating to the work of health professionals. For **questions 1 to 6**, choose the answer (**A, B** or **C**) which you think fits best according to the text.

Write your answers on the separate **Answer Sheet**.

1. The notice reminds staff that patients who are dying

    (A) will need to be prescribed anti-emetics.

    (B) might not need to continue with certain medication.

    (C) should be encouraged to discuss their condition with loved ones.

END-OF-LIFE DECISION MAKING

Remember the five priorities when caring for a dying patient:

1. Recognise that the end of life may be approaching.
2. Communicate with patients, families, carers and staff.
3. Involve patients and those close to them in decision-making.
4. Support the needs of families and carers.
5. Develop an individualised plan of care for the patient.

An end-of-life care plan must ensure the physical, psychological, social and spiritual comfort of the patient, and should strive for the best possible quality of life for the patient's remaining time. This includes prescribing anticipatory medications which can be given as required, falling under the following categories which staff are encouraged to remember as the 'Four As': Analgesia (pain relief), Anxiolytics (anti-anxiety), Anti-emetics (for nausea and vomiting), and Anti-secretory (for respiratory and airway secretions). Any unnecessary medications, such as long-term diabetes control and blood pressure medications can be stopped. A Do-Not-Resuscitate (DNACPR) decision also needs to be made.

---

2. The guidelines inform us that multiple anaesthetics can be used

- (A) to increase the numbing effects.
- (B) to prevent bleeding throughout the procedure.
- (C) to more accurately control how long it will last.

ANAESTHESIA USE AT HARLOW DENTAL CENTRE

At this practice, preference is given to the use of local anaesthetics in combination with conscious sedation.

Many local anaesthetics may be used in order to reversibly block specific pain pathways and/or cause paralysis of muscles. The most commonly used local anaesthetic at the centre is lidocaine - remember that the half-life of lidocaine in the body is about 1.5 to 2 hours. Other local anaesthetic agents include articaine, bupivacaine, prilocaine and mepivacaine. Often, a combination of local anaesthetics may be used, sometimes with adrenaline or another vasoconstrictor to modulate the metabolism of the local anaesthetic and control local bleeding.

Sedation during procedures should mostly be limited to conscious sedation. Benzodiazepines enhance the effect of neurotransmitter gamma-aminobutyric acid (GABA) at the $GABA_A$ receptor. This results in a sedative, hypnotic, anxiolytic, anticonvulsant and muscle relaxant properties.

---

3. The purpose of this memo is to explain

    (A) how to treat multi-resistant pathogens.

    (B) the causes of bacterial infections.

    (C) when to prescribe antibiotics.

For the attention of all medical staff:

Microbial resistance to antibiotics is on the rise and infection with multi-resistant pathogens, such as Clostridium difficile and MRSA amongst others, is becoming more common.

Patients receiving antibiotics are at increased risk of such infections. As such, please be aware of our antimicrobial prescribing guidelines, which ensure that antibiotics are only prescribed with clear, clinical justification; evidence of infection; and/or guaranteed medical benefit.

It is recommended that specimens should be cultured and results obtained before commencing treatment with antibiotics, thus only prescribing the therapy to which the microbe is sensitive. Prescription of broad-spectrum antibiotics should be avoided where possible, as these not only damage the normal bacteria of the human body, but also increase microbial exposure to anti-microbial medications, increasing their potential for developing resistance. Review narrow-spectrum antibiotic prescriptions within 5 days, and broad-spectrum prescriptions within 48 hours.

4.   This guidelines on autism in young people inform us that

   (A)   the disorder is more difficult to identify in patients with ADHD.

   (B)   most children with autism are diagnosed before the age of three.

   (C)   young people with autism are more likely to suffer from other conditions.

AUTISM IN YOUNG PEOPLE

More than 1% of the UK population has an autism spectrum disorder. Signs can vary widely between individuals and at different stages of an individual's development. When children present with other conditions such as ADHD (attention deficit hyperactivity disorder) or other learning difficulties, autism spectrum disorders often go undiagnosed.

In children with autism spectrum disorders, symptoms are present before three years of age but diagnosis can be made after this age too. Individuals with autism spectrum disorder tend to have issues with social interaction and communication, including: difficulty with eye contact, facial expressions, body language and gestures. Often, children with autism spectrum disorders may lack awareness or interest in other children and tend to play alone.

The causes of autism spectrum disorder are unknown but are linked to several complex genetic and environmental interactions.

---

5. The memo reminds all staff to avoid

Ⓐ challenging a patient's criticisms.

Ⓑ handling grievances of a sensitive nature.

Ⓒ recording complaints that are not legitimate.

SUBJECT: FIELDING PATIENT COMPLAINTS

For the attention of all hospital staff:

At County Green Hospital, we endeavour to provide our patients and families with the highest quality of services. Unfortunately, there may be times where performance does not meet expectation. We routinely survey our patients on how we can do better, but members of the treatment team may also be approached with patient feedback, so all employees must be aware of the correct procedure for handling patient complaints. The first step is to listen to what patients have to say and document details appropriately. Whether or not you feel there is a legitimate grievance, it is important to keep a record for later examination. While listening to the complaint, the employee should validate the patient or family member's experience. This does not mean there needs be agreement about the nature of the complaint, but that the employee demonstrates a clear understanding of why the patient or family member might be feeling this way.

---

6. Patients with delirium are more likely to recover quickly if

    (A) kept in a darkened environment.

    (B) staff changes are kept to a minimum.

    (C) treatment ensures they receive adequate rest.

DIAGNOSTIC CRITERIA FOR DELIRIUM

Delirium affects up to 87% of patients in intensive care and is particularly common among the elderly. Delirium can have serious adverse effects and even lead to mortality and must therefore be treated as a medical emergency.

All hospital staff must know how to prevent, detect, and rapidly assess and treat delirium on the hospital wards. Risk factors for developing delirium include: change of environment, loss of vision/hearing aids, inappropriate noise or lighting, sleep deprivation, severe pain, dehydration, drug withdrawal, infections of any kind, recent surgery, and old age. For patients at risk of delirium, think of the mnemonic DELIRIUM which indicates the common causes: Drugs or Dehydration, Electrolyte Imbalance, Level of pain, Infection or Inflammation (such as post-surgery), Respiratory failure, Impaction of faeces (severe constipation), Urinary retention, Metabolic disorder (such as liver or renal failure).

Management requires re-orientation of the patient to where they are and who everybody around them is, as well as re-assurance and a non-confrontational, empathetic approach towards agitated and distressed patients. Please refrain from changing the staff of the medical team responsible for a delirious patient's care, in order to ensure consistency for the patient. Avoid unfamiliar noises, equipment and staff in the immediate vicinity of the patient, and facilitate visits from family and friends as much as possible.

Part C

In this part of the test, there are two texts about different aspects of healthcare. For **questions 7 to 22**, choose the answer (**A**, **B**, **C** or **D**) which you think fits best according to the text.

Write your answers on the separate **Answer Sheet**.

Text 1: Work-Related Stress & Medical Errors

Stress is a term that crops up all too often in modern conversation, used to describe every unfortunate circumstance, every out-of-sequence event, and every foot out of line. What is stress? Most definitions of stress cover any internal or external stimulus which results in a negative response or disturbance in one's physical, social or mental wellbeing. Unfortunately, stress is common, and it can be devastating to people's lives and health when it is maintained over long periods of time, and when when it gains the capacity to overwhelm one's coping abilities and mechanisms.

In the medical profession, daily stress is almost guaranteed. Recently, changes to many healthcare workers' contracts in the UK have resulted in longer and more antisocial working hours, as well as an increased workload, greater bed crises in hospitals and larger budget cuts, so stress levels amongst UK healthcare professionals are on the rise. A 1996 questionnaire study in the Lancet reported that 27% of doctors in the UK believed that the stress they experienced was triggered by poor management, low job satisfaction, financial concerns, and patients' suffering, amongst other factors.

Over two decades later, these problems still exist; some healthcare workers argue that conditions have actually deteriorated. A 2013 report by the British Medical Association stated that over 50% of UK doctors had experienced an increase in work-related stress over the preceding year, in addition to an increase in the complexity of their work. 25% of junior doctors in hospitals also reported a reduced quality of care for patients due to high levels of stress and the pressures put on individual members of staff, with levels of stress exacerbated by longer working hours. In many healthcare jobs, stress is the **elephant in the room**, particularly with junior staff, who may feel unable to voice concerns about their workload. Unfortunately, however, these factors have the potential to lead to medical mistakes, which could be detrimental to patient lives. In such a circumstance, who is really to blame? The overworked medical staff, or the poor management of modern hospitals?

We do not need to look far to examine the effect that stress can have on doctors today. In 2015, Dr Hadiza Bawa-Garba was found guilty of manslaughter after failing to provide life-saving treatment to a patient when needed, resulting in the unfortunate death of a six-year-old child, Jack Adcock. In 2018, this experienced senior paediatrician with a previously unblemished record was struck off the medical register, unable to ever practice again as a doctor. The case of Dr Bawa-Garba infuriated many in the medical profession, as fingers were pointed at an overworked doctor working under immense pressure who was blamed for gross negligence. But who is the truly negligent one in our current healthcare system? While the death of young Jack is extremely saddening, it is important to explore the circumstances around his death in order to prevent such tragedies from reoccurring. On the day of the incident, Dr Bawa-Garba was covering her own workload as well as that of two senior colleagues who were away, across six wards, spanning four floors, with malfunctioning IT software and out-of-order results systems. Did Dr Bawa-Garba make detrimental mistakes? Yes. But one must ask, are we creating a recipe for disaster when we require our medical staff to work under such immense pressures? Could this be one tragic event of many waiting to happen? Such mistakes ruin lives.

Studies have shown that the most common cause of medical errors is the use of heuristics in medical decision-making, leading to bias. Heuristics are shortcuts taken to reach decisions quickly, based on previous patterns of disease and similar cases seen by the doctor. Mistakes are more likely when such shortcuts are used by junior doctors who lack the experience necessary to make such fast decisions accurately. Tversky and Kahneman outlined seven types of heuristics in their 1974 article: Availability heuristics are based on how easy specific diagnoses are to recall, resulting in over-diagnosis of rare but memorable conditions; Representativeness heuristics are based on similarity of patient presentations to previous typical cases, leading to delayed or missed diagnoses in atypical or non-characteristic patients; Anchoring heuristics occur when a diagnosis is based on one piece of information only, leading to rapid conclusions which lack evidence and early diagnosis without consideration of all available information; Confirmation bias occurs when a diagnosis is based on a pre-conceived idea, where the doctor pays attention to the information that supports their theory, and evidence which challenges the diagnosis is consciously or subconsciously ignored; Commissioning bias where a doctor acts too soon rather than waiting to gather and review all the information first; Gambler's Fallacy which is where consecutive patients have the same diagnosis and so the doctor assumes a similar patient who follows must also have the same diagnosis; Fundamental Attribution Error which is the tendency to blame patients rather than their circumstances for their poor health.

Research shows that the best way to avoid medical errors in diagnosis is to consider several hypotheses, known as "differential diagnoses", and investigate **them** all equally until the one with the most supporting evidence is found and agreed upon. Use of heuristics and the resultant flawed decision-making could be prevented by reducing work stresses and pressures on medical professionals. One way to achieve this would be to reduce working hours and shift durations in order to prevent sleep deprivation in medical staff, which is known to hinder focus, thus creating a safer medical environment for both staff and patients.

Text 1: Questions 7 to 14

7. The first paragraph explains that stress

   A is usually caused by a factor than cannot be controlled.

   B is interpreted in various ways by different people.

   C is unusual when it lasts for an extended time.

   D generally impacts people's behaviour.

8. In the second paragraph, doctors are said to claim that stress

   A is often improperly managed by chronic sufferers.

   B could be improved by increasing the welfare budget.

   C generally resulted in their having to work longer hours.

   D was caused by a number of issues including money worries.

9. The writer uses the phrase '**the elephant in the room**' to emphasise the fact that

   A levels of stress experienced by staff has declined.

   B senior staff generally experience less stress than their juniors.

   C many healthcare professionals do not discuss the stress they experience.

   D junior doctors have reported a lower quality personal life as a result of stress.

10. Why does the writer comment on Dr Hadiza Bawa-Garba and her patient Jack?

    A to suggest that doctors are more likely to make significant errors when stressed

    B to outline a scenario where a doctor's concerns about stress were ignored

    C to demonstrate that stress in healthcare professionals is unacceptable

    D to emphasise the impact the death of a patient can have on stress

11. The writer suggests that Jack Adcock's death was partly caused by

    A technology that was out of date and faulty.

    B a hospital ward overcrowded with patients.

    C an insufficient number of nursing team staff.

    D a lack of experience among the clinical team.

12. Why might doctors who use heuristics be at a greater risk of making clinical errors?

    A heuristics are more likely to be used by junior doctors

    B doctors might take too long to complete their tasks

    C doctors might skip over the relevant information

    D the different types of heuristics are confused

13. The writer claims that confirmation bias might cause doctors to ignore relevant information if

   (A) they have recently treated a patient with the same condition.

   (B) they are very familiar with the evidence being presented.

   (C) the patient displays extreme symptoms.

   (D) it does not support their existing theory.

14. What does the word '**them**' refer to in the final paragraph?

   (A) the team of healthcare staff

   (B) a variety of possible causes

   (C) the mistakes in patient care

   (D) a number of different texts

Text 2: Electroconvulsive therapy (ECT)

Electrodes. Wires. Bite Blocks. For many these terms bring to mind a sinister mental asylum and the foreboding image of a patient about to suffer a tortuous electric shock. Literature written in the 20th century did much to criticise this practice, with writers frequently describing electroconvulsive therapy (ECT) as a form of torture, reserved for the most vulnerable members of society. Interestingly enough, ECT has actually been used in the healthcare field for hundreds of years. Before the advent of effective antipsychotic medications, a wide variety of therapies were trialled for serious mental illnesses. One of these involved the therapeutic use of inducing seizures in patients. As early as Benjamin Franklin's (1705 – 1790) time, an electrostatic machine could be used to cure someone of 'hysterical fits'.

Through the 19th century, British asylums began to employ electroconvulsive therapy in a widespread effort to cure diseases of the mind. In the early 20th century, a neuropsychiatrist by the name of Ladislas J. Meduna promoted the idea that schizophrenia and epilepsy were antagonistic disorders, and that precipitating seizures could serve as a potential treatment of schizophrenia. There were several methods used to induce seizures, including insulin coma, seizure-inducing medications (metrazol), and most famously, ECT.

While many of these practices are now seen as barbaric, there were very few options for psychiatric treatment before the development of antipsychotics, mood stabilisers, and anti-depressants. With the rise of these new treatment options came an increase in the public awareness of the often inhuman conditions of electroshock. The revelations resulted in widespread backlash, and the use of ECT therapy began to swiftly decline. However, in the later part of the 20th century, after much debate and research, the National Institute of Mental Health in the US came to a consensus that ECT was both safe and effective when proper guidelines were implemented. In the US today, ECT treatment is routinely covered by insurance for severe and treatment-resistant forms of mental illness.

The exact mechanism of action for ECT is unknown, but there are several hypotheses: Firstly, increased release of monoamine neurotransmitters such as dopamine, serotonin, and norepinephrine; secondly, enhanced transmission of monoamine neurotransmitters between synapses; thirdly, release of hypothalamus or pituitary gland hormones and fourthly, anticonvulsant effect. ECT has several indications, the most notable being refractory major depression, catatonia, persistent suicidality, and bipolar disorder. It is also used in pregnancy as it is effective and does not have the teratogenic effects of some other psychiatric medications. While there are no absolute contraindications, **it goes without saying** that when using ECT, the risks involved will carry more weight with certain patients. Those with unstable cardiovascular conditions, those who have recently suffered a stroke, and those with increased intracranial pressure, severe pulmonary conditions, or a high risk in anaesthesia may not be suitable candidates for ECT. To further explore the appropriateness of using of ECT on specific patients, consider the following case study.

The patient, let's call her Dana, is a 35 year old female who has a history of schizophrenia. She was taken to the hospital by ambulance because her parents found her motionless in her bed, staring blankly, not responding to external stimuli, and not eating or drinking for two days. The psychiatrist caring for her is understandably concerned, because this represents symptoms of catatonia. If Dana does not eat or drink, she may develop life-threatening nutritional deficiencies and electrolyte imbalances. If she does not move, Dana may end up developing a blood clot that could result in a fatal pulmonary embolism. The first-line treatment is benzodiazepines, but in this particular case, there is no improvement in her condition. The psychiatrist decides that that ECT is the next best option. There is the issue of informed consent. Legal jurisdiction handles this differently throughout the world, but if a patient lacks capacity or is too ill to provide consent, a court must provide substitute consent to ensure adequate legal oversight. Once this happens, Dana is medically screened and prepped for treatment.

A course of ECT treatments does not have a standard regimen. Generally, most patients require between six to twelve treatments, but the actual endpoint is determined by the level of improvement. ECT is often given two to three times a week, usually on a Monday/Wednesday/Friday schedule with psychiatric symptoms and testing carried out on a regular basis to monitor progress. Dana starts Monday by being NPO (nothing by mouth) except for any necessary medications. This reduces the chance for aspiration under anaesthesia during the seizure. She will be taken down to the ECT suite where an anaesthesiologist, psychiatrist, and nurse will greet her. She will be placed in a supine position with EEG monitoring to determine the quality of the seizure given. She will have electrodes placed on her head bitemporally, bifrontally, or unilaterally on the right. In this case, given her life-threatening catatonia, we will use the bitemporal position. The anaesthesiologist will then induce anaesthesia, first preoxygenating the patient, then administering anticholinergic agent to reduce oral secretions, anaesthesic medication, muscle relaxation medication, and any cardiovascular prophylaxis as needed.

Once the patient is sufficiently sedated, a brief (0.5 to 2.0 milliseconds) electrical pulse will be introduced at a level determined to reliably cause a seizure. A therapeutic ECT seizure should last at least 15 seconds but no more than 180 seconds. Dana will be monitored for thirty to sixty minutes once **this** has finished, to ensure her recovery. The goal is for further treatments to reduce her symptoms and enable her to eat, drink, communicate, and move again. Of course, there are adverse effects that must be considered. Anaesthesia can cause nausea, aspiration pneumonia, dental and tongue injuries. The seizure itself can cause cardiovascular issues, and fractures in patients with osteoporosis, and can temporarily impair cognition and memory. It is advised that patients do not make any major or financial decisions during or after ECT treatment, and patients must refrain from driving until a few weeks after the last session.

For most patients, one treatment may be all that is needed. For some, continuation of ECT as a single session every couple of weeks may help to prevent relapse. Maintenance treatment for patients with chronically recurring psychiatric illness may also be appropriate. The scheduling of these sessions generally depends on the patient's needs and episodes, sometimes even going on indefinitely. In Dana's case, a few treatments are all that is needed to resolve her catatonia and soon she will be healthy enough to be discharged home with outpatient follow-up for her mental health management.

Text 1: Questions 15 to 22

15. In the first paragraph, the writer mentions the role of 20th century literature in

   (A) informing patients of the side effects of antipsychotic medication.

   (B) preventing the mistreatment of defenceless people.

   (C) increasing the number of patients receiving ECT.

   (D) promoting a negative image of ECT.

16. What do we learn about schizophrenia in the second paragraph?

   (A) It was less prevalent in patients who experienced seizures.

   (B) It had a significant impact on the treatment of epilepsy.

   (C) Many asylums in the UK were not prepared to treat it.

   (D) The medication metrazol could be used to induce it.

17. What did the US National Institute of Mental Health decide in the 20th century?

   (A) Practitioners must follow identical treatment plans when using ECT.

   (B) Patients should be given the right to refuse ECT treatment.

   (C) ECT should only be used as a treatment in severe cases.

   (D) ECT was accepted as a safe treatment for patients.

18. In the fourth paragraph, what idea does the writer emphasise with the phrase **'it goes without saying'**?

   (A) Some women find ECT treatments successful while carrying a child.

   (B) It is well known that some patients will not respond well to ECT.

   (C) Few patients realise that they could benefit from ECT therapy.

   (D) The risks associated with ECT are rarely discussed.

19. In the case study, the psychiatrist decides to use ECT on Dana

   (A) despite Dana's parents' concerns about this type of procedure.

   (B) because the patient expresses a preference for this treatment.

   (C) after treatment with benzodiazepines proves ineffective.

   (D) as she has developed an electrolyte imbalance.

20. In the sixth paragraph, why isn't Dana given food before her ECT treatment?

   (A) to lower the likelihood of anaesthesia-related aspiration

   (B) to reduce the likelihood of vomiting during treatment

   (C) as medication can interfere with the treatment

   (D) as the catatonic state makes eating difficult

21. In the seventh paragraph, what does the word '**this**' refer to?

    (A) a treatment plan

    (B) a seizure caused by ECT

    (C) an abnormal reaction to medication

    (D) an improvement to the patient's condition

22. In the final paragraph, the writer suggests that Dana's treatment

    (A) was complete after only one ECT session.

    (B) will ultimately cure her catatonia using only ECT sessions.

    (C) will continue for a number of weeks before improvement can be seen.

    (D) will consist of two ECT sessions each week for the foreseeable future.

END OF READING TEST

Writing Section

Read the case notes below and complete the writing task which follows.

Notes

Mr. Jacob McCarthy, an 82-year-old, is a patient in the medical-surgical unit of which you are a physician.

Hospital: Jefferson County Hospital, 35 Franklin Street, Knox

Patient Details

  Name: Mr Jacob McCarthy

  Next of kin: Barbara McCarthy (76, spouse)

Admission date: 06 April 2018

Discharge date: 26 April 2018

Diagnosis: Right below knee amputation (BKA) status post right foot diabetic ulcer

Past medical history: Benign prostatic hyperplasia, diabetes mellitus Type 2 (non-compliant with medication), age-related dementia, essential hypertension, peripheral vascular disease, osteoarthritis

Social background: Retired construction worker

         Wife primary carer

         Moderate cognitive impairment

         Needs assistance with medication and activities of daily living (ADL's)

On admission:	Long history of noncompliance with diabetic medication.
	Admitted for infected right diabetic foot wound of at least two weeks, did not notice injury → diabetic neuropathy.
	Obvious signs – gangrene, pus, abscess.
	Fever, chills, R foot non-weight bearing.
	Blood cultures positive for gram-positive cocci.
Medical progress:	Given IV antibiotics, vascular surgeon consulted to assess wound.
	Recommended BKA.
	Surgery performed without complication.
	Transitioned to oral antibiotics and opiates.
	Currently afebrile – wound is clean, dry, intact.
	Requires assistance for ADLs + wheelchair for mobility.
Nursing management:	Monitor surgical site for infection/drainage.
	Check for fever/chills + other signs of infection.
	Encourage oral fluids, nutrition.
	Assist with ADLs and mobility.
	Change dressings daily.
	Ensure good urination and bowel movements.
	Frequent turning – avoid decubitus ulcers.
Assessment:	Good progress made, pain under control, no further infection noted.
	Blood cultures now negative.
	Mobility severely reduced after amputation – requires assistance for ADLs and routine care.
Discharge plan:	Discharge to Skilled Nursing Facility for acute care and physiotherapy.
	Can reassess later for stability with home nursing vs. long-term care facility.
	Continue antibiotics and pain medication.
	Will need to follow-up with vascular surgeon in 2 weeks.
	Of note, wife wanted discharge to home in her care – physiotherapy and occupational therapy assessment indicate this would not be a safe discharge.

Medical Writing Task

Using the information given in the case notes, write a discharge letter to Dr. Shannon Meccam, Medical Director of Knox Skilled Nursing Facility, 25 Harrowfield Avenue, Knox.

In your answer:

- **Expand the relevant notes into complete sentences**
- **Do not use note form**
- **Use letter format**

The body of the letter should be approximately 180 – 200 words.

Nursing Writing Task

Using the information given in the case notes, write a transfer letter to the receiving nurse at the skilled care facility, Shannon Meccam, Knox Skilled Nursing Facility, 25 Harrowfield Avenue, Knox.

In your answer:

- **Expand the relevant notes into complete sentences**
- **Do not use note form**
- **Use letter format**

The body of the letter should be approximately 180 – 200 words.

Please record your answer on this page.

_____

_____

_____

_____

_____

_____

_____

_____

_____

_____

_____

_____

_____

_____

_____

_____

_____

_____

_____

_____

_____

_____

Please record your answer on this page.

Speaking Section

You have 5 minutes to complete the tasks in the candidate card, while talking with a patient.

Read the candidate card now, and take 2-3 minutes to prepare for your conversation.

Medical Task Card Set 1

CANDIDATE CARD NO. 1	MEDICINE
SETTING	Suburban Clinic
DOCTOR	You are speaking to a 50-year-old patient who has come to find out the results of a core needle biopsy (removal of cells and tissue) from the lymph node of a swelling in their right armpit. He/she has a history of cancer (previous thyroid), but has been in remission for two years. The test results indicate Hodgkin lymphoma and further tests are needed to determine the staging (the spread of the cancer).
TASK	• Find out what result the patient is expecting from the test. • Find out how much information the patient wants today. • Sensitively, explain the test results (e.g. the biopsy indicates Hodgkin lymphoma (cancer of the lymph nodes) and further testing is needed, like CT scans, to assess staging – the spread of the cancer, etc.). Check for understanding and reassure if needed. • Explain that the stage is unclear, so further advice will be given later. • Summarise the information given and find out what further information is needed.

ROLEPLAYER CARD NO. 1	MEDICINE

SETTING	Suburban Clinic
PATIENT	You are a 50-year-old who has recently found a lump in your right armpit. A sample was taken and you have come to find out the results. You have had thyroid cancer before and have been in remission for two years. You are worried that it is cancer again.
TASK	• Explain that you are not sure what the results are, but you are worried that the lump is cancer. • Explain that you have had cancer before, so if it is cancer, you want all the information possible. • Be a little shocked and worried. Find out what the prognosis is and if you have to stop working. • Be unclear why this has happened to you. Explain that you would like to read more information on the disease.

You have 5 minutes to complete the tasks in the candidate card, while talking with a patient.

Read the candidate card now, and take 2-3 minutes to prepare for your conversation.

Medical Task Card Set 2

CANDIDATE CARD NO. 2	MEDICINE
SETTING	Suburban General Surgery Practice
DOCTOR	A 42-year-old patient has come to see you for a post-operative appointment after having an open cholecystectomy (removal of the gallbladder with one incision) performed five days ago for acute cholecystitis (inflammation of the gallbladder). Recovery was uncomplicated, However, he/she is worried about their future and keen on understanding why this occurred and what changes must be made to avoid this happening again.
TASK	• Find out how the patient has been recovering. Go over a recovery timeline and explain the level of physical activity he/she should be able to perform (4-6 weeks to fully recover; light exercise only).
	• Discuss the patient's current diet and best practices now that he has had a cholecystectomy (avoid high-fat/spicy foods, eat small meals to start with, track diet, etc.).
	• Explain possible future complications (e.g. post-cholecystectomy syndrome) and the signs of symptoms to look out for and when to go to the Emergency Department (ED) (e.g. if acute pain in the abdomen/diarrhoea.
	• Give the patient an estimation of how long they will need to have follow up appointments for (once every two weeks for six weeks).

ROLEPLAYER CARD NO. 2	MEDICINE

SETTING Suburban General Surgery Practice

PATIENT You are 42 and recovering from acute cholecystitis (inflammation of the gallbladder, often caused by gallstones) that began one week ago. You were discharged from the hospital after an open cholecystectomy (removal of the gallbladder with one incision) five days ago. You are unsure how much physical activity is appropriate and do not want to risk tearing out any stitches. You also want to know what this means for your diet, and if there is anything you need to watch out for.

TASK

- Explain your concerns about physical activity and find out how long you need to wait before you can return to work.

- Explain that you live alone and don't like to cook, so your diet is primarily pre-packed frozen meals or fast food. Ask the doctor what could happen if you do not follow the recommended diet?

- Ask what are some future complications to be aware of?

- Ask how often should you schedule follow-up appointments with the clinic?

You have 5 minutes to complete the tasks in the candidate card, while talking with a patient.

Read the candidate card now, and take 2-3 minutes to prepare for your conversation.

Nursing Task Card Set 1

CANDIDATE CARD NO. 3	NURSING

SETTING	Suburban Clinic
NURSE	You are speaking to a parent of a 4-year-old boy, Max, who has Autism Spectrum Disorder (ASD) and has come to see you for dietary advice. He is globally delayed (mentally, physically and emotionally) and displays difficult behaviours at the childcare centre he attends (e.g. becomes upset if asked to sit with other children at meal times, etc.).
TASK	• Explore the parent's perception of the problem.
	• Find out how the parent is structuring meal times at home.
	• Create some realistic goals with the parent (e.g. provide regular meals and snacks – every 2-3 hours, change the mealtime environment – gradually move from the TV to the table, etc.).
	• Find out what other services the parent needs (e.g. speech therapy – oral motor development, integration aide for the childcare centre, support group, etc.).

ROLEPLAYER CARD NO. 3	NURSING

SETTING	Suburban Clinic
CARER	You are the parent of a 4-year-old boy, Max, who has Autism Spectrum Disorder (ASD) and is a very fussy eater and will only eat baby food, smooth yoghurt and mashed potato with you at meal times. You are worried that he is not getting enough nutrients, and that he is not progressing socially with his peers. He becomes angry at the childcare centre when asked to eat with the other children.
TASK	• Explain that the problem started as a response to a viral infection at 2 years old, but has now become a habit. Max only eats mushy food with you in front of the TV.
	• Ask the nurse if Max will develop a vitamin deficiency.
	• Describe mealtimes: you have to prompt Max to eat while you hold the spoon, and Max is angry if you change the brand of food. He often eats late in the day, and self-feeds sweet biscuits.
	• Be resistant to any big changes in routine. You could probably only change one thing.
	• If asked, you would like to see a speech pathologist and attend a support group, but the childcare centre doesn't have funding for integration aides.

You have 5 minutes to complete the tasks in the candidate card, while talking with a patient.

Read the candidate card now, and take 2-3 minutes to prepare for your conversation.

Nursing Task Card Set 2

CANDIDATE CARD NO. 4	NURSING

SETTING	Hospital
NURSE	You are speaking to a 90-year-old patient who was recently admitted to hospital due to vomiting, nausea and abdominal pain, which was later diagnosed as acute pancreatitis. The doctor has ordered no food by mouth (NPO), so a nasogastric (NG) tube has been inserted. Intravenous (IV) fluid with potassium chloride (KCI) and his/her pain medication, meperidine (Demerol), have been ordered.
TASK	• Explain the reasons for the NG tube (to alleviate pain from eating, and to allow feeding until nausea and vomiting subside). Likely to stop after two days. Check that the patient understands your explanation. • Tactfully explain why the NG tube is inserted with more detail (e.g. large meals require additional work by the pancreas for digestion, the inflammation stops this, and causes pain, etc.). • Reassure the patient about the further testing (CT scans – non-invasive, relatively safe, involves x-rays, able to detect complications e.g. necrosis – tissue death). • Validate the patient's concerns but explain the low levels of radiation (e.g. less than from a flight). Reassure the patient that the tests are needed.

ROLEPLAYER CARD NO. 4	NURSING
SETTING	Hospital
PATIENT	You are a 90-year-old who was recently admitted to hospital due to vomiting, nausea and abdominal pain, which was later diagnosed as acute pancreatitis. You have a tube in your nose and haven't been given any food. You are anxious and don't understand what is happening to you and want answers from the nurse.
TASK	• Ask the nurse why you have a tube in your nose and haven't been allowed to eat solid food.
	• Explain that you still don't understand why you can't eat. The tube is uncomfortable, and you miss your favourite foods.
	• When asked, explain that you want to know what happens next. You don't know what tests you will have to do, and you are worried.
	• Continue to be worried about the tests; you don't want radiation and you just want to go home. Eventually be reassured.

Answers

Listening

Part A: Questions 1 to 12

1	up the stairs
2	barking
3	lying down
4	(dirty) green
5	feverish
6	COPD
7	smoker
8	allopurinol
9	knees
10	(blue) inhaler
11	cholesterol
12	penicillin

Questions 13 to 24

13	stuck (in it)
14	watering
15	swollen
16	concentrate
17	fluorescein eye stain
18	infection
19	(numbing) eye drops
20	corneal abrasion
21	antibiotic eye drops
22	healing ointment
23	ibuprofen
24	bright light

Part B: Questions 25 to 30

25	**A**	be transferred from the Emergency Department
26	**B**	whether his communication issues will improve
27	**A**	explaining how to use them correctly
28	**C**	the availability of a medicine.
29	**C**	the importance of providing adequate emotional support to patients
30	**A**	identifying the patients at greatest risk

Part C: Questions 31 to 36

31	**B**	mistake the illness for something else.
32	**B**	proximity to new people.
33	**C**	He was trying to finish his assignments.
34	**A**	the illness progresses rapidly.
35	**B**	patients do not seek treatment quickly.
36	**C**	take precautions to prevent others from becoming ill.

Questions 37 to 42

37	**A**	suffer from untreated health problems.
38	**C**	reduces the likelihood of the provider being injured.
39	**A**	to ensure the patient understands what is being said.
40	**B**	acknowledge the patient's emotions
41	**B**	maintain the patient's trust by being realisable.
42	**C**	be encouraged to explain what caused their reaction.

Reading

Part A: Questions 1 to 20

1	C
2	B
3	A
4	D
5	A
6	B
7	arterial saturation
8	magnesium sulfate
9	allergies
10	life-threatening
11	reversibility testing
12	smoking
13	daily
14	every hour
15	in severe cases
16	children
17	warn ICU
18	peak expiratory flow rate **OR** PEFR
19	a whistling sound
20	a peak flow meter

Part B: Questions 1 to 6

1	B	might not need to continue with certain medication.
2	C	to more accurately control how long it will last.
3	C	when to prescribe antibiotics.
4	A	the disorder is more difficult to identify in patients with ADHD.
5	A	challenging a patient's criticisms.
6	B	staff changes are kept to a minimum.

Part C: Questions 7 to 14

7	**B**	is interpreted in various ways by different people.
8	**D**	was caused by a number of issues including money worries.
9	**C**	many healthcare professionals do not discuss the stress they experience.
10	**A**	to suggest that doctors are more likely to make significant errors when stressed
11	**A**	technology that was out of date and faulty.
12	**C**	doctors might skip over the relevant information
13	**D**	it does not support their existing theory.
14	**B**	a variety of possible causes

Questions 15 to 22

15	**D**	promoting a negative image of ECT.
16	**A**	It was less prevalent in patients who experienced seizures.
17	**D**	ECT was accepted as a safe treatment for patients.
18	**B**	It is well known that some patients will not respond well to ECT.
19	**C**	after treatment with benzodiazepines proves ineffective.
20	**A**	to lower the likelihood of anaesthesia-related aspiration
21	**B**	a seizure caused by ECT
22	**C**	will continue for a number of weeks before improvement can be seen.

Writing

Medical Sample Response

Dr. Shannon Meccam
Medical Director
Knox Skilled Nursing Facility
25 Harrowfield Avenue
Knox

26/04/2018

Dear. Dr. Meccam,

Re: Jacob McCarthy (aged 82)

Mr McCarthy was admitted on 6 April 2018 with a right diabetic foot ulcer. A vascular surgeon was consulted, who recommended that he undergo right below the knee amputation, which was performed without complication.

Following surgery, Mr McCarthy was placed on IV antibiotics and pain medications, these have been successfully transitioned to oral antibiotics. His wound has been healing well and his repeat blood cultures have been negative.

Mr McCarthy is now stable, and can be discharged to your facility for further care. He will continue to need assistance for ADLs as well as a wheelchair for mobility. His surgical site should be assessed for infection and his dressings must be changed daily. He should also receive frequent turning to prevent pressure ulcers.

Of note, his wife wanted him to be discharged back to his home under her care; however, we feel that given his dementia and decreased mobility following the amputation, this would not be considered a safe discharge. Our physiotherapy and occupational therapy staff agreed with our assessment. We feel that after some time at your facility he may show sufficient improvement to return home.

If you have any queries, please contact me.

Yours sincerely,

[185 words]

Nursing Sample Response

Shannon Meccam
Nurse
Knox Skilled Nursing Facility
25 Harrowfield Avenue
Knox

26/04/2018

Dear Nurse Meccam,

Re: Jacob McCarthy (aged 82)

Mr. McCarthy was admitted on 6 April 2018 with an infected right diabetic foot ulcer and positive blood cultures. Past medical history includes benign prostatic hyperplasia, diabetes mellitus Type 2, dementia, hypertension, and peripheral vascular disease.

A vascular surgeon was consulted, who recommended a right below the knee amputation, which was performed without complication. Following surgery, Mr McCarthy was placed on IV antibiotics and pain medications which have been successfully transitioned to oral administration. His wound is healing well and repeat blood cultures are negative.

Mr. McCarthy is now stable for discharge to your facility. He will continue to need assistance for ADLs and a wheelchair for mobility. His surgical site should be assessed for infection, with daily dressing changes. He should also receive frequent turning, to prevent pressure ulcers.

Of note, his wife wanted him to be discharged back to their home under her care; given his dementia and decreased mobility following the amputation, physiotherapy and occupational therapy staff did not believe this was a safe discharge plan. After some time at your facility, he may show sufficient improvement to return home or a decision made for long-term care placement.

If you have any queries, please contact me.

Yours sincerely,

[199 words]

Listening Script

Part A

N: I'm going to give you the instructions for this test. I'll introduce each part of the test and give you time to read the questions.

This test has three parts. In each part you'll hear a number of different extracts. At the start of each extract, you'll hear this sound: ---***---. You'll hear each extract ONCE only. Remember, while you're listening, write your answers on the question paper. At the end of the test, you'll have five minutes to transfer your answers on to the separate answer sheet.

Part A. In this part of the test, you'll hear two different extracts. In each extract, a health professional is talking to a patient. For questions 1 to 24, complete the notes with information you hear. Now turn over and look at the notes for extract one.

PAUSE: 5 SECONDS

N: Extract one. Questions 1 to 12.

You hear a foundation doctor talking to a recently admitted patient called Roy Miller. For questions 13 to 24, complete the notes with a word or short phrase.

PAUSE: 30 SECONDS

---***---

F: So, Roy, I see from your notes you've been admitted because of shortness of breath. Can you tell me more about that please?

M: Yeah... well it started last week. I noticed that getting up the stairs was more of an effort and I found that I had to pause on the way, to catch my breath. I did used to get a little out of breath, but it's definitely gotten worse. I normally manage to go shopping with my wife and we walk to the shops and back. I'd generally have to have a little rest, but now, everything is just taking me longer. I feel weary, you know? And I've got this cough, it's like a barking thing that I just can't shift. It's worse at night when I'm lying down and I get a bit wheezy. I'm just really tired because it keeps me awake for most of the night. My wife has been sleeping in the spare room because it's keeping her awake... I've also sort of been bringing up things when coughing... Without being too graphic, it's quite thick, its a sort of dirty green colour, I suppose. It wasn't like that at the beginning of last week, it was just clear but over the last couple of days I've noticed it's changed colour and I'm coughing up a lot more. My wife was starting to get worried so she made me an appointment with our doctor and then he sent me here.

F: OK Roy. Do you have any other symptoms?

M: Yeah, I was really hot yesterday and I thought it was because the heating was on, but my wife hadn't turned it on. Then the next minute I was shivering. I guess I'm feverish?

F: It sounds like you've been really suffering. Have you got any other medical conditions?

M: Well I was diagnosed with this lung condition last year, I've forgotten the name of it, hold on . . . . . CO, CO, hang on I'll get it, COPD, is that it? Well anyway they told me that my lungs weren't working as well as they could be because I used to be a smoker, but I quit about 6 years ago. To be honest I think it was because I worked in the mines and it was really dusty. Either way I've got it and it makes me a bit breathless but nothing like this. Oh and I also get gout from time to time and I take something called allopurinol or something. I've also got arthritis in my knees but that's just because of my age so I just put up with that.

F: You mentioned taking allopurinol. Are you on any other medication?

M: Well, the doctor gave me inhalers, and I'm using those. I'm getting better at taking them because I found it a bit confusing at first. I've started to take my blue inhaler a lot more over this last week because I've been so breathless. I take the stuff I mentioned before, a statin for my cholesterol and then the odd paracetamol when my arthritis starts to play up. I don't really like taking pills but if it keeps me going then it's worth it . . . Also, I'm allergic to penicillin. I get an awful rash all over my body and it's so itchy whenever they give it to me. Don't give me any of that!

F: We won't Roy. You mentioned you live with your wife, are you both managing at home?

M: Oh yes, we still get around the town to get our shopping and see the family. The stairs are starting to get a bit much now so we're thinking about moving into a bungalow, but we haven't started looking yet.

F: OK that's good. Have you got any ideas as to what might be going on?

M: Well I think it might be a chest infection because it's just getting worse. I just want to start feeling better.

F: Of course Roy, it does sound like that might be the case, but we'll start doing some tests to make sure and begin treatment.

PAUSE: 10 SECONDS

N: Now look at the notes for extract two.

Extract two. Questions 13 to 24.

You hear an optometrist talking to a patient called Marsha Samarina. For questions 13 to 24, complete the notes with a word or short phrase.

PAUSE: 30 SECONDS

---***---

M: Hi, Marsha Samarina? I'm Dr Kulshaw. I understand that you've been experiencing some issues with your left eye?

F: Yeah that's right.

M: Okay, are you able to tell me a bit about what's been happening?

F: Yeah sure. So, last Friday was our office party, and so I was out quite late, and I'd had a couple of glasses of wine. Anyway, when I came home I must have been a bit reckless taking out my contact lenses. I didn't notice anything then, but when I woke up in the morning I had this pain in my left eye... it felt like there was something stuck in it. Also, I had a headache, I'm not sure if that's because I was straining my eyes. My eye was also watering loads, it was kind of like what happens when you chop up onions. Anyway, I thought I'd just sort of keep blinking, and whatever was in my eye would work its way out... so, well I did that for a bit, but I was getting more and more worried. I went to ask my roommate if she could see anything in my eye, and she said my eye was swollen and she thought we should go to the hospital and get it checked out. So we went to the ED... Thankfully my roommate was able to get the day off work, so she drove me there. The pain was also so terrible that I couldn't concentrate. I don't know what I'd have done without her help.

M: Ah, okay... so what happened when you went to the hospital?

F: So we waited around at the ED for a bit, and then I was seen by a GP... umm... I told him about the pain, and how I thought I had something stuck in my eye so he opened my eye and tried to see if there was anything in there that shouldn't be. It must have been quite difficult for him to see anything, so he did a fluorescein eye stain test... then he took me to a dark laboratory room to look into eyes with one of those, um, microscope things. When he still couldn't find anything he seemed to think that it could be an infection. That's when I started panicking!

M: And after that, you were referred to an optometrist?

F: Yes, that's right. They sent me to this department after that, and the optometrist used some numbing eye drops on me– I was incredibly thankful to her for that! My eyes felt better very soon afterwards. Then she looked at my eye, and because I wasn't squinting from the pain anymore, she could see that there was a corneal abrasion, she said that I must have scratched it when I took my contacts out the night before.

M: I see, so can you tell me how you've been treating your eye at home?

F: Yes, she told me not to wear my contact lenses until this follow up, and she pre-scribed me a couple of things... I'm using the antibiotic eye drops she gave me – I put those in in the mornings and evenings... and the other thing she gave me is really horrible to use, it's a healing ointment, but it feels gross in my eye so I just use it once a day. Unfortunately, they couldn't give me any of their pain relief to take home, so I've just been taking ibuprofen when it hurts.

M: And how's your eye feeling now?

F: Much better, thanks. It still hurts when there's bright light though, and I wasn't sure if that was normal? The optometrist said it would take quite a while to heal, so I guess I need to hang on a bit longer?

M: Yes, at this point it will most likely still be recovering. Do you mind if I take a close look at your eye now? If you can just take your glasses off...

PAUSE: 10 SECONDS

N: That is the end of Part A. Now, turn over and look at Part B.

PAUSE: 5 SECONDS

N: Part B, questions 25 to 30. In this part of the test, you'll hear six different extracts. In each extract, you'll hear people talking in a different healthcare setting.

For questions 25 to 30, choose the answer A, B or C which fits best according to what you hear.

Now look at Question 25. You hear two doctors discuss the transfer of care for a patient. Now read the question.

PAUSE: 15 SECONDS

---***---

M: Hello, Dr Salvos? This is Dr Broderick from the Emergency Department. I'm calling you with regards to an admission to the hospital medicine service.

F: Right, yes. Hello Dr Broderick… I'm the admitting physician for hospital medicine… Umm, Can you tell me more about the patient, and why he needs to be admitted from the emergency department?

M: Sure… So the patient is a 68-year old man with a past history of CHF, DM2 and a chief complaint of shortness of breath for three days. Chest X-Ray shows a right lower lobar pneumonia. His vital signs are normal but his BUN is 36.

F: I see… It sounds like he meets CURB-65 criteria for an inpatient admission. Have you started him on any medications in the emergency department?

M: Yes, we have given him supplemental oxygen and started him on breathing treatments. He will also be getting empirical antibiotic coverage. If there are any other orders you would like me to place, let me know and I'll do so.

PAUSE: 5 SECONDS

N: Question 26. You hear a speech pathologist talking to the wife of a patient who has recently suffered a stroke. Now read the question.

PAUSE: 15 SECONDS

F: I just don't really understand why my husband can't speak properly anymore. Is it a result of brain damage?

M: Problems of this type are a result of damage to the brain, yes, but it's important to note that these issues haven't affected your husband's intelligence.

F: No, of course. I know it's still him. It's just frustrating when we can't talk like we used to. Will he get better eventually?

M: Your husband has shown improvement already, and we're confident that this will continue with regular sessions and practice. Patients tend to show the greatest change within the first six months, which is why we've planned such an intensive schedule for him during this time. We're confident that we'll see great strides in your husband's condition over the coming months.

PAUSE: 5 SECONDS

N: Question 27. You hear a trainee doctor asking a senior colleague about chest tubes. Now read the question.

PAUSE: 15 SECONDS

F: I'm still just a bit unsure about chest tubes… I was hoping you might be able to give me a bit more information?

M: Okay, sure. So you know about the three chambers on the chest tube, right?

F: Yep. There's the collection chamber, the water seal chamber, and the wet or dry suction regulator.

M: Right. So as the air from the pleural space passes though the water-seal chamber, you should see gentle fluctuation in the water every time the patient breathes. This is called tidaling. If you notice that tidaling is no longer present, the tubing may be kinked or obstructed, or the patient's lung may have re-expanded.

F: Ahh, okay

M: You should also make sure the chest drainage unit remains below the level of the patient's chest at all times.

PAUSE: 5 SECONDS

N: Question 28. You hear a pharmacist talking to a customer about pain relief. Now read the question.

PAUSE: 15 SECONDS

F: Hello, can I help you?

M: Yes. I get terrible back ache, and my friend said you could give me some codeine for it?

F: Do you have a prescription from your doctor?

M: No. But I don't want the full strength stuff. I only need the weaker one. Y'know, they mix it with ibuprofen or paracetamol, so it's not as strong.

F: Ah okay. Well, first of all, there's been some research done recently that suggests that low dose codeine doesn't offer much more pain relief than paracetamol or ibuprofen alone. We're not actually authorised to provide codeine without a prescription anymore, so I'd recommend picking up some alternative pain relief from the first aisle by the front door.

N: Question 29. You hear a trainee nurse receiving feedback from his tutor. Now read the question.

F: How do you feel you handled the patient's concerns?

M: Well, I think I was okay. Maybe I wasn't as confident as I could've been? I'm still quite nervous about advising patients. I guess I just need more experience to gain confidence.

F: Maybe, but I actually don't feel that was an issue for you. Do you think there's anything else you could've done for the patient during your examination? You could, perhaps, have tried to be more reassuring, rather than just stating the facts? Sometimes patients need to feel like their anxieties are being heard.

M: Yeah... I actually think I did cover this with the patient, though. He talked through his concerns while I was examining him.

F: It's not enough for the patient to say they're feeling worried, you have to show that you're listening, and reassure them that you're working with their best interests in mind.

N: Question 30. You hear two doctors planning their patient-care schedule Now read the question.

M: We have twenty four patients in total to see today, across two bays... and unfortunately, we only have four staff members... I think we should divide ourselves into two teams. Would you agree?

F: Absolutely! Also, I think we should see patients according to their National Early Warning Score, that way, we'll get through all those who have urgent requirements before lunch... then we can be sure that the most pressing investigations are performed earliest, and the sooner we get those organised the better. Phlebotomists will be coming to the ward at around half one, so any blood forms should be given to them then.

N: That is the end of Part B. Now, turn over and look at Part C.

N: Part C, questions 31 to 42. In this part of the test, you'll hear two different extracts. In each extract, you'll hear health professionals talking about aspects of their work.

       For questions 31 to 42, choose the answer A, B or C which fits best according to what you hear.

Now look at extract one. Questions 31 to 36.

You hear an interview with a physician called Dr Matthew Leach, who's talking about meningitis.

You now have 90 seconds to read questions 31 to 36.

PAUSE: 90 SECONDS

---***---

F: Hello everyone, I'm here with Dr. Matthew Leach, an expert on infectious disease, who's going to tell us about meningitis. Thank you for being with us today, Dr. Leach. Can you tell me more about the disease?

M: Sure. Well first off, not everyone who is exposed actually develops meningitis, but there are some common symptoms to look out for in those that are at risk. It can be quite difficult for patients to realise they have meningitis in the early stages, as the symptoms can lead them to believe that they are developing the flu, they'll simply feel tired and achey for a few days… As this infection develops, patients may then notice a sudden onset of fever, headache, and in particular, neck stiffness. Other possible symptoms include nausea or vomiting, confusion, sensitivity to light, no appetite or thirst, or even a skin rash. If left untreated, bacterial meningitis is very dangerous, quickly progressing to seizures, shock, and even death.

F: That sounds pretty serious. You mentioned that certain people may be at risk. Which people are the more likely to develop meningitis?

M: Well, there are many causes of meningitis, but one of the most severe is caused by the bacteria *Neisseria meningitides*. The bacteria are spread by respiratory droplets, and are often seen in college students. This is largely because of the sudden change in their lifestyle. College students, particularly those who live on campus, are exposed to a hotbed of different infections that they haven't previously encountered – all these kids from different parts of the US and the rest of the world get together, live in small dorms with each other, go to parties… all that close contact really is a breeding ground for infection.

F: Okay, that makes sense. Now, can you tell us about a specific patient who had this type of meningitis?

M: Of course. I treated an 18 year old man in his first year of college who was living in the dormitories. There was a flu going around, and he started to feel the same symptoms. He was working hard to try to complete a couple of important essays before the deadline, and he planned to delay going to the doctors until he had submitted them. Soon after the initial symptoms, however, his roommate found him in severe pain and feverish, and brought him to the emergency department where we diagnosed meningitis. We took a sample of spinal fluid, but started him on antibiotics before we got the results back.

F: So, you mentioned that you started antibiotics before you got the spinal fluid test results back. Can you tell me why?

M: Right. As I mentioned, there are many causes of meningitis, like viruses, funguses, parasites, and bacteria. However, it can take some time to determine the exact cause, and waiting for the answer without treatment will make the patient worse. Instead, we use the patient's presentation, age, and our determination of the most likely cause to start antibiotics that would kill many of the causes. Once we get the results back on the cause, we can change the antibiotics to be more specific. By doing this we don't delay treatment, and are able to reduce the chance of complications.

F: Ah right I see… so how is your patient doing now after being treated? Will he experience any long term after-effects?

M: Well, he is currently doing much better. He responded well to antibiotic treatment and regained his mental state within a few days. Unless the patient has a disease of his immune system, meningitis is unlikely to recur. Because this patient had some delay before seeking treatment, he may still have some side effects, but it will take some time to see what long term effect it will have on him. Bacterial meningitis requires urgent medical treatment, and can cause serious complications such as hearing loss, memory difficulty, brain damage, gait problems, or kidney failure.

F: Well, let's hope he makes a full recovery. Aside from seeking immediate medical treatment, what advice can you give to our listeners today about bacterial meningitis?

M: So, first off, there is a vaccine that is effective at preventing this disease, so anyone in close contact with a large group of people, such as those living in a military base or on a college campus, should ask their doctor about it. Finally, if you have not had the shot and have spent a lot of time with someone who is later diagnosed with meningitis, wear a mask to prevent spreading the bacteria, and go and see a doctor immediately. There are medications that can reduce your risk of developing meningitis, and getting treated immediately will reduce your risk significantly.

PAUSE: 10 SECONDS

N: Now turn over and look at extract two. Questions 37 to 42.

You hear a clinical psychiatrist called Dr Evalina Houghton discuss treatment for agitated patients in an emergency setting.

You now have 90 seconds to read questions 37 to 42.

PAUSE: 90 SECONDS

F: Hello everyone! My name is Dr Evalina Houghton and in my presentation today I'd like to discuss an issue that I deal with daily, de-escalating agitated patients in an emergency setting. To provide some perspective on the issue, most patients who enter the hospital do so via the emergency department (ED). Many won't have received medical treatment yet, and that can make it more likely for these patients to become agitated. This can be exacerbated by their medical condition, a psychiatric illness, or other stress factors. Given the chaotic and crowded nature of the ED, it's imperative that we identify agitated patients early and apply non-physical de-escalation techniques as soon as possible.

The provider who is going to initiate the de-escalation process should make sure that they create a considerable amount of space between themselves and the patient, and make sure that no one else is closer to the patient than they are. This not only gives the patient space, but also keeps the provider safe in the event of attempted physical violence. Ideally, both the patient and provider should also be able to leave the area without the other blocking their exit. Body language and tone of voice convey overall emotional state to a patient, so providers should remain outwardly calm throughout the encounter.

When speaking to the patient, you should start by introducing your name and role in the team. You should determine how the patient prefers to be addressed and err on the side of being respectful. Use short sentences and simple vocabulary to enhance understanding. Leave a suitable amount of time between statements to allow patients to process what is being said – sometimes repetition and enunciation may be necessary. Eye contact should be intermittent, so the patient does not think you're staring, and verbal responses should be calm without any hint of insults or challenges. Only one provider should interact with the patient, as multiple speakers can confuse an agitated patient.

When the patient speaks, it's important to identify what their wants and feelings are, even if they may be impossible to address at this time. Try to consider things from the patient's perspective. Although they may be suffering under a particular delusion, such as paranoia, try to understand how the patient might feel or react if that delusion happened to be true. While we do not want to endorse these delusions, it's important to find common ground. For instance, if the patient is agitated because they think they are being followed, the provider can agree with the general principle, saying something like "I understand that your suspicion of other people can make it hard to get the treatment you need here." It is also okay for a provider to agree that while they may not be having the same experience as a patient with an obvious delusion, they can believe the patient is having that experience and reacting to it.

In addition, patients should be encouraged to make choices, in order to give them a sense of control over the current situation and defuse their overall aggressiveness. These choices should be realistic, however, and deliverable, as unfulfilled promises may backfire and irreparably damage the therapeutic alliance. Some of these choices can include medications to help calm the patient. A good way to state this is "It's important for you to stay calm so we can talk. Can we provide you some medication to help you feel less anxious?" Offering patients a choice between different medications or routes of delivery may also provide a feeling of control to the patient.

Lastly, when the crisis is over, a key technique is debriefing both the patients and staff on how the situation went. The patient, now calm, may be able to provide more insights on what they were thinking and how they were feeling at the time. The provider can discuss coping skills or alternative options in order to prevent another aggressive incident in the future. It is also important to talk to staff as well, to gain any third-party feedback on the provider-patient interaction, what was appropriate, what helped de-escalate the patient, and any other changes that could be made to ensure patient, staff, and bystander safety.

These techniques can be applicable to a wide variety of patients in numerous settings, they're not just restricted to the emergency department. Our hope is that providers will be able to deescalate patients safely and effectively without having to resort to the use of physical or chemical restraints, which should be considered only when all other approaches have failed.